CHIROPRACTIC PHYSIOLOGY

A Review of Scientific Principles
as Related to the
Chiropractic Adjustment
With Emphasis On
Bio Energetic Synchronization Technique

M.T. Morter, Jr., B.S., M.A., D.C.

B.E.S.T. Research, Inc.
1000 W. Poplar
Rogers, Arkansas 72756

Chiropractic Physiology
M.T. Morter, Jr., D.C.

Copyright © 1988 by B.E.S.T. Research Inc.

Printed in the United States

Library of Congress Cataloging-in-Publication Data
Morter, M.T.
        Chiropractic Physiology.

        1. Chiropractic.   2. Sensorimotor integration.
3. Spinal adjustment — Physiological aspects.   I. Title.
[DNLM: 1. Chiropractic.   WB 905 M887c]
RZ242.M67   1988   615.5'34   88-70369
ISBN   0-944994-01-6

*The quality of a person's life
is in direct proportion to their
dedication to excellence*

Vince Lombardi

CONTENTS

FOREWORD

Every doctor has patients who have received conventional chiropractic, physical therapy, and have been to virtually every type of doctor. We see the patient, pull out our magic bag of tricks and our favorite modalities, and the patient feels better, leaves and comes back two days later feeling at least as bad if not worse than the first time we saw them. This pattern is frustrating for both the therapist and the patient.

The beauty of the Bio Energetic Synchronization Technique is that it deals with many levels, including the emotional factors that perpetuate pain.

Historically, the resurgence in the use of stimulation in improving physiological functioning dates back to Melzack and Wall, who published the gate control theory of pain. Melzack and Wall performed a very interesting historical review on the treatment of pain. Most interesting were the cases where there was no physiological correlate to the presence of pain. For example, many patients who are amputees will not only feel the "phantom" limb in space, but will also experience excruciating pain at the extremity. Every known pathway mediating pain had been cut in these unfortunate patients, (cutting off afferent input). Interestingly, even complete myelotomies were unsuccessful. Only anesthetizing the sensory cortex provided partial pain relief; this left Melzack and Wall with the absurd conclusion that pain was not carried by peripheral nerve, but that pain was a central phenomenon stored in the nervous system and that a memory-like mechanism was involved.

In summary, patients with "phantom" limb pain suffered from the pain because of error in central read-out. The central read-out could be modified much more easily by gentle tapping of the amputated stump, by gentle vibration, or by whirlpools. The exciting part about Melzack and Walls' theory was that it predicted that very subtle stimuli delivered to the muscle afferents would be much more capable of producing pain relief than neurosurgical intervention.

The Melzack and Wall hypothesis predicted the usefulness of electrical stimulation. Receiving less fanfare, however, is the prediction that very mild stimulation of the muscle afferents provided almost anywhere in the body would produce long-lasting relief from chronic pain. And from their design of the nervous system and the circuits involved, this is undoubtedly the case. Entire movements in physical therapy have evolved using stimulation such as sheep's wool, light vibration, pressure, stretching, and even subtler modalities in order to stimulate muscle afferents.

The Bio Energetic Synchronization Technique goes several steps beyond. It utilizes the gate control theory which Dr. Morter discovered independently since he has been performing the Bio Energetic Synchronization Technique for twenty years. It utilizes light touch and is totally non-invasive. *It also treats the areas opposite to the painful area, and has independently noted that treating the painful area first, just like in acupuncture, just like in any form of electrical stimulation, makes the pain worse!* The advantage to Bio Energetic Synchronization is not only its surprising efficacy but the fact that it is totally non-invasive, requires no tools, except a heart, a mind, and two hands, and can be performed anywhere. It is perfect for emergency situations. The purpose of the Bio Energetic Synchronization Technique is to alter afferent input just like the other techniques, but it does so in a non-invasive way.

I am not easily impressed. I studied at McGill University when Melzack and Wall came up with their famous gate control theory, and it takes a lot to convince me. I am a skeptic at heart, but I am always willing to learn new techniques to help a greater number of people. I have a Ph.D. in neurophysiology and have five years of experience studying the effects of stimulation on the nervous system of animals. Because of my deep conviction that stimulation of the nervous system produced results that were virtually miraculous in brain damaged animals, I decided to get my M.D. and went into rehabilitation medicine because I felt that the animal research could really benefit human beings. Most of my patients have spinal cord injuries and are told that they are paralyzed and nothing can help them. A smaller number has intractable pain due to scoliosis and other skeletal deformities. Dr. Morter showed me how I could help my patients beyond the modalities that they were receiving. Immediately obvious was the release of muscle tension and spasticity in patients with chronic spinal cord injury. One patient who has suffered a very serious shoulder problem for which he had been hospitalized and received morphine improved dramatically after one treatment, and his pain disappeared after the second time. He had failed all previous modalities. I use the technique on staff who have pulled their muscles and they are immediately better. But the most astounding case was a lady with scoliosis I had treated for six months and who kept returning. In one 8-minute treatment we threw away her shoe lift and she walked without an antalgic gait. The pain relief has lasted several weeks. That was much better than I can perform after six months of various kinds of therapy including acupuncture.

It seems quite obvious that the nervous system does have a memory and the patient cannot relax poor muscle spasms because his nervous system has not learned to do so. Some trauma, whether it is emotional or physical, has produced a defensive reaction in muscle spasm. Unless we replace that memory with another one indicating that it is safe to relax the muscles, the patients will never improve. I think that every pediatrician, and every practicing physician should know how to use the Bio Energetic Synchronization Technique. The world would be better off.

Judith B. Walker, M.D., Ph.D.

Dr. Walker is Director of Medicine at the Walker Institute, a center for the treatment and rehabilitation of central nervous system trauma and intractable pain in Pacific Palisades, California.

ACKNOWLEDGMENT

One of the primary themes of this book is that we are stimulus/ response beings. Not only is our internal functioning a response to stimuli, the actions we take in our daily lives are responses to stimuli generated by the various people and circumstances we encounter.

The circumstances surrounding the writing of this book is a case in point. For many years, I had intended to investigate the relationship of scientific principles to the consistent results that are achieved by the Bio Energetic Synchronization Technique (B.E.S.T.). However, as is often the case, other projects captured my attention. It was not until circumstances produced a specific stimulus that I turned my attention to scientific literature that provided the basis for this work.

With this in mind, I want to acknowledge the governing authorities in the chiropractic profession in general and the Texas Board of Chiropractic Examiners in particular for the impetus they supplied in spurring me on to achieve this long-held goal.

In addition, my appreciation goes to the many doctors of chiropractic who have attended my seminars and who have adopted B.E.S.T. into their practices, and to the thousands of patients who accept B.E.S.T. as their principal health care system. Each of them has contributed, in their own way, to bringing this study to print.

To my children, my sincere appreciation for their continued loyalty, support, and encouragement. And, particularly, to my wife, Marjorie, goes special credit for her selfless dedication to both B.E.S.T. and our family.

INTRODUCTION

This paper reviews the unique position chiropractic holds in the health care field, offers a view based on accepted scientific principles of the impact of chiropractic adjustments on the many anatomical and physiological systems of the body, and presents an overview of the Bio Energetic Synchronization Technique as a chiropractic procedure that utilizes chiropractic and other scientific principles to directly address the source of interference.

Comments regarding the material contained in this report are welcome and should be addressed to B.E.S.T. Research Inc., 1000 West Poplar, Rogers, AR 72756.

M.T. Morter, Jr., B.S., M.A., D.C.

1

SYNOPSIS OF CHIROPRACTIC AND EVALUATION OF THE BIO ENERGETIC SYNCHRONIZATION TECHNIQUE

OBJECTIVES OF BIO ENERGETIC SYNCHRONIZATION TECHNIQUE

- Provide comprehensive health care in accordance with chiropractic principles.

- Consistently effect improvement in patient's chief complaint, homeostatic balance, sensory-motor integration, and vertebral alignment through chiropractic manipulation.

- Improve overall health of patients in the most safe, effective manner possible.

- Include in technique procedures only actions that are of benefit to the patient.

THESIS

Bio Energetic Synchronization Technique is a chiropractic procedure that allows vertebral position and visceral function to be improved by updating present physiology (sensory awareness) to suit present need.

Bio Energetic Synchronization Technique is a method of introducing non-traumatic stimuli to the highest level of the central nervous system. These stimuli initiate physiological responses that facilitate the body's homeostasis-seeking nature to achieve lasting auto corrections by the musculoskeletal and other systems.

Bio Energetic Synchronization Technique further proposes:

1. A definite quantifiable relationship exists between structure and function.

2. Subluxations are the result of muscular motor response.

3. The sensory system responds to internal and external stimuli and in turn stimulates impulses that initiate motor activity.

4. Interference in the central nervous system above the level of the intervertebral foramen (IVF) can cause structural imbalance and functional disorder.

5. The vast majority of stimuli that initiate sensory responses originate in memory.

6. Improved vertebral position, visceral function, and muscle tone will occur when the efferent system is allowed to accurately respond to external and internal stimuli presented by either present sensory input or memory.

TENETS APPLICABLE TO ALL CHIROPRACTIC TECHNIQUES

The following statements are basic tenets of the science of chiropractic that are applicable to all techniques.

1. The human body:

    a. is comprised of a network of integrated systems,

    b. must be considered as a totality greater than the sum of its parts,

      c. maintains its vitality through an integrated, unified stimulus-response action, and

      d. never makes a mistake.

2. Every manifestation of human existence is a response to at least one internal or external stimulus.

3. Every chiropractic adjustment affects the entire body.

4. Integrity of the spine is essential in maintaining proper structure-function relationship and normal nerve impulse transmission.

5. A subluxation is an osseous disrelationship associated with abnormal nerve function.

6. The body seeks homeostasis by adapting, via stimulus-response action, to internal and external stimuli.

7. Every response of the body is always correct for the stimulus even though the response may appear to be antagonistic to homeostasis.

8. Cerebellar impulses can be inappropriate to present need, cause paravertebral muscle imbalance, and thereby affect vertebral position.

9. Impulses will travel both proximally and distally from the point of nerve stimulation.

10. Internal stimuli affecting homeostasis are acted on through the hypothalamus.

11. Conscious thought is controlled by the cerebral cortex.

12. Conscious awareness that allows conscious physical reaction to environment is controlled by the thalamus.

13. Subconscious activity, of which the person is unaware, is subcortical.

14. Subcortical responses are never judgmental.

15. Subconscious activity is controlled by the hypothalamus even though it may be influenced by the thalamus.

16. Unconsciousness indicates inability to react voluntarily to external stimuli even though subconscious physiological functions continue.

17. Most impulses that reach the cortex pass through the thalamus which acts on all stimuli from conscious awareness.

18. The sensory system responds to stimuli that indicate a threat to homeostasis.

19. The sensory system initiates corrective impulses to which the motor system responds.

20. The central nervous system contains substantially greater numbers of sensory fibers than motor fibers.

21. The motor system can act as a servomechanism which functions according to patterns provided by the sensory areas of the nervous system, including the brain.

22. More than 99% of all incoming sensory information is discarded by the brain.

23. Sequential patterns for a particular activity can be stored in subconscious memory engrams and recalled to activate a motor system response.

24. Ninety-nine percent of present physiology is controlled by memory engrams which are stored in the subcortical areas of the brain.

25. Voluntary and involuntary muscles are largely controlled by memory engrams.

26. Vertebral position is determined by muscle balance and tone.

27. Vertebral position is dictated by subcortical response to information from muscle spindles and Golgi tendon organs.

28. Subcortical muscle response patterns may be updated by vertebral adjustments.

29. Subcortical muscle response patterns can be updated by specific tactile stimulation of paravertebral areas.

30. The great majority of current physiology is controlled by past experience (engrams) which may contain compensations for a prior stress.

31. Internal and external sensory information along with memory input are all compared and integrated in response to any new physical position, i.e., recumbent.

32. The adrenal response may be initiated by engrams of past stressful experiences.

33. The adrenal response (General Adaptation Syndrome) includes the stages of (1) awareness, (2) adaptation or facilitation, and (3) exhaustion.

34. The adrenal response (fight-flight) can be activated when the hypothalamus is stimulated by a real or imagined stress.

35. Any force (light or heavy) is instantly appraised by the entire nervous system and affects the entire body.

36. Traumatized muscles may assume and maintain a spasmus condition appropriate for the demands of that emergency.

37. When the patient has assumed the horizontal position, the necessity of sustaining previous defensive physiology is no longer appropriate.

38. Accurate current sensory information must be made available to the coordinating centers of the nervous system to allow corrective responses to occur.

39. An updated memory engram will dictate a corrected vertebral position, therefore, when the righting reflex is re-engaged, the corrected normal position will be manifest.

40. Updating memory engrams to show that a crisis position is no longer appropriate will permit normal response thereby allowing a sustained corrected vertebral position.

OBSERVATIONS

1. Primary interference occurs in the brain.

2. Properly aligned vertebrae allow afferent as well as efferent nerve impulses to be transmitted freely.

3. For accurate impulses to be received by the motor system, interference must be removed from all levels of the central nervous system.

4. The thalamus-hypothalamus complex is most susceptible to interference due to its highly sophisticated integration of sensory information.

5. A subluxation can be the result of a correct response to a past stimulus which is no longer appropriate.

6. Subluxations occur following trauma as vertebrae, mandated by memory engrams, inappropriately remain in the position associated with the trauma.

7. Forceful adjustments affect the response of the muscle spindles and the Golgi system as well as the defense mechanism.

8. Ninety-nine percent of a patient's physiology may be responding to a stress reflex from a past experience.

9. Inappropriate physiology (including vertebral position) may be the result of stored memory patterns (engrams) dictating responses that are inappropriate for current internal and external stimuli.

10. If response pattern correction is not achieved at high brain levels, subcortical impulses will re-create the subluxation.

11. Abnormal vertebral position can be corrected indirectly as well as directly.

12. Vertebral position can be improved directly through the sensory system by updating memory engrams thus permit-

ting subcortical areas to recognize that a position based on past stimuli may no longer be appropriate for present intent.

13. Homeostatic equilibrium is possible when complete integration of the body is indicated by equal leg-lengths and equal arm-strength.

COMMENTARY

The preceding statements represent underlying principles that contribute to successful adjustments in all chiropractic techniques in general and the Bio Energetic Synchronization Technique in particular. Although some of the concepts may not be recognized as being instrumental in core chiropractic adjustments, careful study of the physiology of the adjustment reveals that any manipulation of the body will either directly or indirectly stimulate response.

2

CHIROPRACTIC — A UNIQUE HEALTH CARE DISCIPLINE

UNIFIED THOUGH DIVERSE

Chiropractic has recently successfully withstood an eleven-year-long assault against its professional validity — the recent ruling of a federal court represents a tremendous victory for the profession. This litigation can serve as a graphic reminder to us that, in our efforts to regulate chiropractic, we must not place ourselves in the same culpable position in which the medical establishment found itself, and from which it could not retreat and eventually became entrapped.

As the growing number of patients who look to chiropractic illustrates, our profession is not only surviving, it is flourishing. The chiropractic profession alone provides the drug-free, non-invasive, holistic health care and maintenance that knowledgeable health-conscious people not only want but demand.

Although the confrontation with our detractors is not over, we know what the outcome will be as long as we are true to our philosophy and keep our house in order. To be sure, chiropractic, after a mere 93 years, has survived its infancy and is moving into the more accident-prone stage of the toddler; we are taking the knocks and spills that are a part of growing up and reaching maturity. As with most youngsters, we are now, for the most part, suffering self-inflicted wounds — wounds that are the result of rapid growth and, perhaps, of losing sight of our collective professional goal of helping sick people to get well and healthy people to stay well. If we persist, instead, on focusing our corporate energy on infighting centered around the variations in the methods used to reach this goal we, as a profession, become much more vulnerable to attack and much less cohesive in our defense.

There is no reason for chiropractic to be divided against itself. As a profession, we have proved that we can help people achieve and maintain health. Each individual chiropractor can cite personal incidents of seemingly miraculous results — there is no question that chiropractic works, and that it works through the professional tenets that were developed by D. D. Palmer nearly 100 years ago. The chiropractic philosophy is the foundation upon which the profession is united. While each chiropractor treasures his own interpretation of D. D.'s legacy, it is generally agreed that chiropractic

- treats the whole person rather than merely symptoms,

- recognizes a structure-function relationship that influences total health,

- is a method of health care administered by use of hands, primarily upon the spinal area,

- removes obstructions that impede the flow of nerve impulses,

- is a drugless, non-surgical alternative health care discipline,

- advocates that the power that made the body can heal the body, and

- treats the cause, not the effects, of disease.

Chiropractic has an enviable record of treating the cause of physical distress and of achieving positive results. As long as the profession collectively continues to focus on goals, continues to develop and to explore how and why overall health can improve when bones move, and seeks to establish methods to evaluate scientifically that we, in fact, do what we say we do, chiropractic will not only survive but it will gain even greater momentum.

Throughout the profession, we use the phrase "chiropractic is a science, art, and philosophy." The philosophy of chiropractic sets it apart from other health care systems such as conventional medicine, homeopathy, and osteopathy. Chiropractic is a health care system devoted to considering and treating the patient as a whole entity rather than as animated symptoms. In chiropractic, our patients *have* digestion problems, our patients *are not* digestion problems. As a whole, the profession recognizes that a proper relationship between skeletal structure and physiologic function is essential to relieving symptoms and to allowing the body to heal itself.

THE INNATE CONCEPT

Chiropractic is one of the few well-established modern health care philosophies that recognizes and approaches the body as a self-regulating, self-healing, integrated organism. An almost universally accepted concept in the chiropractic community is that an Innate Intelligence guides the body in adapting to both internal and external environmental changes in order to achieve homeostatic balance. The axiom that the power that made the body can heal the body has been an underlying premise of chiropractic since its inception.

Although the character of Innate has been discussed and disputed throughout the active profession and in chiropractic colleges, its existence as a cradle of physiological repair is generally affirmed. D. D. Palmer stated in *The Chiropractor's Adjuster,* "Innate's existence and consciousness are not dependent upon its body, no more than we are on the house we live in. It is invincible, cannot be injured or destroyed by material changes. It is invulnerable, is not subject to traumatic or toxic injuries, is not subordinate to material substance." Innate is a basic philosophical premise of chiropractic that is defined in many ways. As in describing any intangible (beauty, happiness, grief, pain) the idea of Innate can be portrayed in many ways, yet this diversity of expression does not negate the existence of the abstract concept.

B. J. Palmer wrote for the *Science of Chiropractic,* Vol. 1, 1917, p. 44, "Chiropractors adjust displacements of the bones, relieve pressure from nerves so that they can perform their functions in a normal manner. Then Innate can and WILL do the rest." This statement by one of the founders of chiropractic emphasizes two of the planks in the philosophical platform: chiropractic provides the means through which bones can move; and, chiropractic removes interferences in the nervous system.

Having recognized the inborn authority of Innate in healing, we can move from the philosophical realm to a more verifiable arena of cause and effect, i.e., stimulus/response manifestations. Randomness has little place in our well-ordered universe. Everything that happens in the human body is a response to at least one stimulus. It is not necessary that we understand precisely the sequence of events that takes place between the stimulus and response; we need only accept that a plan exists and the body will express a response to that plan in keeping with its Innate Intelligence. Whether we use the term Innate, Superconsciousness, Universal Intelligence, God, Ultimate Power, Natural Law, or Mother Nature, the concept "the power that made the body can heal the body" is firmly held by the vast majority of chiropractors.

SEPARATING ART FROM PHILOSOPHY

It is safe to say that our professional house shares much common ground in the philosophy of chiropractic; it is no secret that it is divided by vast canyons and that strong feelings separate differing attitudes about how these philosophies can or should be implemented to benefit patients. Yet, if chiropractic is to survive and grow, we must not only recognize our common ground but also be open-minded and flexible enough to appreciate the validity of other points of view. In his book *The Chiropractic Story*, Marcus Bach, Ph.D., a leading lay authority on chiropractic, observed the potential for corporate professional self-destruction over forty years ago, and addressed his concern in his comments on the need for unity in the profession. In describing his impression of the profession and its members at an annual convocation at Palmer School of Chiropractic in the early 1940s attended by about 2000 enthusiastic followers of D. D. and B. J. Palmer, Dr. Bach wrote: "Chiropractic was here to stay and the only thing that could ever defeat this new science and art of healing would be chiropractic itself."

Our differences lie not in the area of the philosophy of chiropractic but in the area of the art of chiropractic. It is universality of agreement on the most effective means of applying these philosophies in the day-to-day practice of treating patients that is lacking. We are in general agreement as to our goals and purposes — the primary objective of chiropractic is to remove interference from the nervous system and to restore health to our patients; we are not in agreement as to the details of the medium with which to meet these goals. At present, vertebral adjusting is the primary procedure used to meet our goals; however, as with any art form, it is the artisan who selects the method with which he is most comfortable that will achieve his aims. If the procedure selected does not produce the results he wants for a particular work, he will either modify his procedure or change to a different method in order to produce the desired outcome.

Differences concerning methods are most apparent between the two primary factions of the profession commonly referred to as "straights" and "mixers." There are those who hold strictly to a literal interpretation of D. D. Palmer's concept that chiropractic is *limited* to the "science and art of correcting abnormal functions by hand adjusting, using the vertebral processes as levers." In the other camp, there are those who honor and follow this precept as the foundation for advancing chiropractic art and science through study, research and application of methods based on additional information.

Disciples of both of these schools of thought have usually been successful in applying their particular art to improve the health and comfort of thousands of patients. It is apparent, however, that limiting chiropractic strictly to hands adjusting vertebrae will not satisfy the needs of all of the patients who come to us for help. If it worked *in every instance*, chiropractors would not have seen a need for adaptations in their procedures. Since 1895, many subtle and some radical variations on the original chiropractic theme have evolved to provide a wide scope of techniques that are used independently or in combination. There are those who practice "straight" chiropractic who have incorporated small deviations into their practice, while other chiropractors who have been schooled in several techniques may use mechanical or electronic devices that seem more appropriate to an individual patient's specific needs. Some adaptations of adjusting techniques have been developed as a means of both achieving more favorable results for the patients and easing physical stress or trauma of both the patient and doctor.

Unfortunately, although enthusiasm and feeling toward given techniques generally run high, neither "straights" nor "mixers" emphasize that their particular technique shows more consistent or verifiable results than do other techniques.

It is vital that our profession, individually and collectively, keeps in mind that the primary goal of chiropractic is to serve the best interest of our patients. Chiropractic is for patients. Although most chiropractors realize a comfortable income from application of their art, this is a by-product of helping patients, relieving pain, and providing effective health maintenance care. Chiropractic was initiated to benefit mankind, not to stimulate chiropractors to heated philosophical or methodological debate. If the profession is to fulfill its commitment to patients to provide the best holistic health care possible, the primary area of concern must be to continue to develop chiropractic procedures that will benefit each and every patient and to establish standardized methods of evaluating the results of all procedures — traditional or innovative.

There is no question that adjusting a vertebra usually brings about favorable results. Many theories have been advanced as to why adjustments are effective, and many techniques are available to accomplish vertebral realignment that will remove nerve impingement. Chiropractic professionals are in general agreement that when pressure is removed from nerves at the intervertebral foramen, relief from both pain and disease will follow. Even the most skeptical antagonists cannot deny that positive results are usually achieved by chiropractic adjustments. It is this impressive record of a high percentage of successful treatments that has perpetuated the chiropractic profession and philosophy.

As chiropractic continues the tradition of aiding patients, we, as a profession, are now secure enough to be able to investigate realistically the effectiveness of a given technique. We can even entertain the thought that perhaps there may be explanations not previously advanced that account for the successes of specific techniques.

Each technique can point with justifiable pride to its own achievements in providing patients symptomatic relief and improved health. Favorable clinical results have been the foundation upon which chiropractic has survived. We never want to give up our heritage merely for the sake of courting the acceptance of others, nor need we relinquish our heritage in order to progress. But progress we must. And to progress, we must constantly be aware of the need to remain flexible in our attitudes and to maintain the open-mindedness we had as enthusiastic students. Our professional "mind" is equally as subject to stagnation and closure as is our individual mind if we refuse to look at and thoughtfully consider a perspective different from the one we first recognized. It is not necessary to wholeheartedly embrace every newly encountered school of chiropractic thought any more than it is necessary or desirable to unhesitatingly follow every different religious concept that comes along. There is a mental "neutral zone" that allows for genuine open-minded inspection of unfamiliar ideas without predetermined acceptance or rejection of those ideas.

In his book, Dr. Bach quotes B. J. Palmer as addressing the issue of rigidity in thinking during one of their dinner conversations (p. 163): "... in your traveling among various cultures you must have found, as I have, that there is no greater virtue than adaptability and no worse sin than being bound by inflexible convictions."

THE FRAGILE PEDESTAL OF CHIROPRACTIC SCIENCE

We have now reached the point where we must examine the source and validity of our current conviction that chiropractic is indeed a science. Do we, in fact, achieve positive results consistently enough to claim true scientific standing? Are our results reproducible? Can we regularly document results through pre-treatment and post-treatment x-rays and laboratory analyses as well as by observations of symptomatic improvement? Since chiropractic claims to treat cause (the source of illness) rather than effect (the symptoms of illness), are we willing to subject this claim to the scrutiny of standardized evaluations?

Our mission is to help sick people get well and our track record shows that we have had a high degree of success in doing this. We can improve our health-restoring success rate by finding out why there has been inconsistency in our results rather than by concentrating on perpetuating only those procedures that have the longest history in the profession. Chiropractic was not born full-grown any more than was any other science, nor has chiropractic yet realized its full potential. Ongoing investigation into how the total body is affected by an adjustment is essential. Chiropractic is designed to help mankind, not just one kind of man — the chiropractor who practices only hands-on-spine adjustments. The measure of chiropractic must be taken by evaluating results, not form.

Additional hard questions can be raised: Can a science be based solely on clinical observation as chiropractic is now? If not, do we, as yet, have a science? Certainly no other science could stand on such a fragile pedestal. Chiropractic can be a valid, genuine science. A science is a systemized body of knowledge. "Science" implies that systematized procedures obtain consistent results; a procedure that works 100% of the time as verified by accepted standards of evaluation is a science.

The scientific mind is an inquiring mind; it is not satisfied with subjective evaluations — opinion and theory can serve as a springboard for scientific study, but for the scientific mind, conclusions and evaluations must be based on quantifiable, objective information. Science, as with any other aspect of life, is vital — ever moving and growing. A science that does not accept the challenge to progress becomes dogma. Progress and movement are synonymous with change, and change can imply uncertainty that some find threatening to either their peace of mind or their cherished beliefs. However, scientific investigation, when carried out systematically, can not only evoke change, it can also strengthen existing tenets and practices.

Clinical observations can serve as a basis for instituting scientific investigation of just what it is we do when we adjust a vertebra. However, clinical observation can tell us whether or not a given procedure works — it cannot tell us how or why it works. Clinical observation shows the effect of an adjustment; it does not give us the cause of the response that will indicate whether the adjustment will have a lasting effect or is merely a temporary palliative. Only by scientifically evaluating quantitatively verifiable data can we evaluate our healing art.

STANDARDS OF EVALUATION

Our heritage bases chiropractic on a structure-function relationship; misaligned vertebrae cause interference with nerve transmissions which results in physiological problems and disease — this is a fundamental tenet that all chiropractors can accept. This premise establishes a base on which to build standards of evaluation for chiropractic that will assure a degree of uniformity in the health care we provide.

With this base established, we must define the criteria for evaluating the results of treatment no matter what technique is used. The first criterion for judging the effectiveness of any technique would be that structural changes following adjustments will be demonstrated more than just *occasionally*, they will *usually* be evident and verifiable. Structural changes can be observed through x-rays taken to conform to consistent standards relative to time intervals and technical precision that will verify patient improvement. The technique should have such a high success rate that on those occasions that the technique doesn't work — when the adjustment doesn't hold — at least one collateral component can be identified as the factor that negated the holding power of the adjustment.

The second criterion would recognize that chiropractic also affects organic function — blood pressure, kidney function, and overall homeostasis — and can substantiate this claim with laboratory findings. Systemic physiology should be improved by chiropractic treatment regardless of the technique involved. Accurate laboratory analysis of blood and urine can demonstrate specific results following certain procedures. However, if the results are less favorable than expected, the reason for failure must be explained. For instance, if the results of treatment of a patient for a bladder irritation are less favorable than anticipated, it may be that the patient has continued to consume large quantities of coffee despite advice to substantially reduce the amount. Under these conditions, the irritation is unlikely to respond to treatment and the reason for the lack of response can be cited.

The third criterion for evaluation addresses the reason most patients come to a chiropractor's office in the first place — relief of symptoms. Valid chiropractic procedures must effect improvement in the patient's chief complaint.

Using these criteria as the basis for evaluation of our professional performance, a protocol can be established to evaluate how the goals of each criterion (structure-function relationship, organic function improvement, and symptom relief) are met. Specific parameters can be defined to assure consistency and quality of performance within the profession. By adopting a system of this nature, each technique will be judged by the same measure rather than by "brand loyalty."

Our colleges of chiropractic could play an important part in standardizing evaluations by using the criteria outlined. Faculty and students alike can undertake scientifically sound research to determine, in an impartial open-minded arena, the effectiveness of various core curricula as well as any new or innovative techniques. We would then have evidence of reproducible results that constitute true science.

There is no question that chiropractic produces results; we learned in college why we get these results. We might also consider that it may be possible — just possible — that there are other physiological factors involved that we have not previously recognized as major determinants in achieving positive results. Accepting this possibility in no way detracts from or diminishes the significant achievements of chiropractic. Reasons and results are unrelated — both can stand alone. We must not be blinded to the successes of any techniques simply because the methods do not fit within the framework of our personal reasoning, belief or perspective.

Standardization of technique should not be the goal of the profession. We can, however, legitimately look to standardizing ways of evaluating whether or not we actually accomplish what we say we can accomplish to improve patients' health. The route taken (the art) to reach a given destination is a matter of personal choice and conviction; the fact that we have arrived at that destination can be verified objectively.

Technique is an art form, a personalized method of achieving particular goals based on clinical results and scientific premises. Part of a doctor's healing skills and effectiveness are due to his rapport with patients, and all patients do not respond equally as well to all doctors. All chiropractors would not — and should not — adopt a single technique. However, as a profession we should be open both to expanding our concepts of chiropractic techniques and to scientifically assessing the consistency of our results.

EXPANDING CONCEPTS

In expanding our concepts of chiropractic, we certainly are not sailing into uncharted waters. In *Chiropractic Economics*, September/October 1981, page 128, Drs. Jenness and Toftness offer some conclusions of their scientific studies "... the primary source of nerve dysfunction occurs in the brain rather than in the spinal cord...." They recognized that our concepts must be enlarged. Dr. Joseph J. Janse, writing in the Jou*rnal of Manipulative and Physiological Therapeutics*, Vol. 1, No. 3, September 1978, also recognized the importance of the sensory system in regaining and maintaining normal physiological function.

In 1895 D. D. Palmer moved a bone and the patient's hearing was restored. Certainly, this was not the first time a bone had been moved, but this one observation served as the springboard for chiropractic. We are all familiar with the story of Isaac Newton using his observation of the falling apple as the catalyst for the discovery of the principles of gravity. Again, this certainly was not the first time anyone had seen an apple fall. Both of these observations were the beginning of developments that have had a major impact on man's world. Neither observation marked the end of further investigation. In his book, *The Stress of Life* (McGraw Hill Book Co., revised edition 1975), Hans Selye, M.D., noted researcher and authority on stress, puts this concept into perspective: "Man can advance from observation to wisdom in many ways — through instinct, for instance by way of faith, intuition, or art. But if the gap is to be bridged by science, the subject of observation must first be clearly defined and measurable."

B. J. Palmer, in the *Science of Chiropractic*, Vol. 1, 1917, page 12, states, "... innate mental impulses control the vital functions... asleep or awake. Conscious or sub-conscious. Cortical or cerebellar." He also noted that disease is caused by either too little or too much energy. So not only a founding father, but past and current researchers of our profession leave the door open to investigation, recognizing that chiropractic was not born fully developed. We can expand our horizons, enlarge our concepts, and establish chiropractic as a scientifically founded and verified healing profession without discarding any of our heritage.

3

A SCIENTIFIC VIEW OF THE CHIROPRACTIC ADJUSTMENT

THE POSITIVE RESULTS OF CHIROPRACTIC

Chiropractic is results oriented. We have seen that chiropractic adjustments bring about symptomatic relief as well as improvement in homeostasis. We have also presented the challenge that, perhaps, the adjustments used to effect these results have been effective for reasons in addition to those generally put forth. Any chiropractor who has been in practice for more than two days has learned that each patient is an individual with his or her own particular physical structure, anatomical and emotional characteristics, life style, and perceptions. This same chiropractor also knows that different patients who have similar complaints for which they receive similar treatment do not invariably respond in a similar manner. Questions raised by observing such diversity of response might be, "What are the unseen factors in the adjustment process that could account for dissimilar responses in apparently similar situations?" Or, simply, "Why are positive results not reproduced every time an adjustment is given?" The material that follows is intended to propose answers, drawn from scientific sources, to these questions.

As with any science, chiropractic must be able to effect reproducible results that can be evaluated by relatively standardized criteria. Accepted clinical methods should be those that achieve positive results. The particular technique used in obtaining the desired results is secondary to achieving our collective goal of restoring, promoting, and maintaining the health of our patients.

Scientific texts set forth principles of physiology that illustrate how chiropractic procedures have brought about improvement in patients' health for nearly 100 years. Authorities in physiology, neurology, biochemistry and other disciplines present information which, when carefully analyzed, explains the reasons chiropractic procedures can usually achieve positive results. These same sources explain why adjustments bring relief to some patients but others expressing similar symptoms experience no improvement. This valuable information is available to us in scientific textbooks used in leading chiropractic and medical schools. Throughout this discussion, reference will be made by author's name and text page number to passages from *The Textbook of Medical Physiology*, Fifth Edition, by Arthur C. Guyton, M.D., published by W.B. Saunders Company, Philadelphia, 1976, and *Medical Physiology*, Vol. II, edited by Vernon B. Mountcastle, M.D., published by C.V. Mosby Company, St. Louis, 1968, as well as other authors.

RELATING PHYSIOLOGY TO THE ADJUSTMENT

A science can be described as a systematized body of knowledge with a corresponding procedure to follow that will lead to consistent results. In general, chiropractic falls short of qualifying as a science under this description since results are not consistent. In addition, as we have often been reminded by the medical profession, our results have not been substantiated. If we say that the structure-function relationship of the body is the basis for chiropractic science, we should be able to consistently bring about structural changes which can be substantiated through x-rays.

Scientific research has already proved chiropractic; however, this research does not prove that a pinched nerve is the cause of all disease. Science can prove that there is an *association* between a pinched nerve and disease — it has not proved that this is a cause and effect. Science has shown how chiropractic addresses physiological dysfunction that can cause disease, and scientific premises can prove what happens in an adjustment. By relating physiology to chiropractic tenets, new avenues are opened for investigation into why and how chiropractic adjustments bring about positive clinical results, including structural improvement, and further research is stimulated into how we can achieve these results more consistently.

Chiropractors learn in school what happens when a bone is moved although the full implications of the principles involved may not be understood. When a vertebra is moved back into alignment, the flow of nerve energy out of the IVF is improved. This would imply that signals coming out of the IVF determine the lasting effectiveness of the adjustment. However, we will see that the sensory information that goes *into* the IVF determines whether or not an adjustment will have a positive, lasting effect. The information that goes to the brain is more crucial to achieving a lasting adjustment than is the information that comes *from* the brain. Information that goes *to* the brain causes the impulses coming *from* the brain to stimulate the motor system to respond in a particular manner.

We shall see that the body's reaction to an adjustment is far more important to maintaining a new vertebral position than is the actual adjustment, and that the sensory nerves going into the IVF, are primarily responsible for maintaining the new vertebral position. It is important that the information being transmitted to the motor system by the higher levels of the central nervous system be appropriate to the present need, not to past experiences.

There are several points that are pertinent to relating scientific premises to chiropractic adjustments.

Vertebrae are bones, and bones are moved by skeletal muscle action. Vertebrae also form joints, and skeletal muscle action is involved in joint movement. However, abnormal vertebral position cannot be consciously corrected. This inability to consciously control some skeletal muscles is illustrated by patients who perceive that they are consciously relaxing specific muscles but the muscles actually remain taut and contracted. Patients cannot consciously totally relax all skeletal muscle tension. The skeletal muscles involved in holding a vertebra in either a subluxated or corrected position are controlled by a *subconscious* center of the brain.

SENSORY INFORMATION AND MEMORY

The nervous system that controls both conscious and subconscious activities can be divided into two general branches: afferent fibers that direct nerve impulses to the brain, and efferent fibers that direct nerve impulses from the brain. Most chiropractic procedures are based on the assumption that the information coming from the motor system of the brain determines the function of organs, position of bones, and tone of muscles. However, this efferent system assumes a secondary role to sensory input in maintaining vertebral repositioning and homeostatic function. The motor side of the nervous system is involved in sending impulses to organs to elicit responses of improved glandular secretion (autonomic), or to muscles to bring about improved muscle cooperation that will accomplish structural homeostatic symmetry. All body language — responses communicated through terms such as structure, organ function, leg length, and other physical signals — is an expression of the motor aspect of the nervous system.

Guyton points out (page 626, *Information, Signals and Impulses*) that "The primary function of the nervous system is (a) to transmit information from one point to another and (b) to process this information so that it can be used advantageously or so that its meaning can become clear to the mind."

The sensory system is responsible for gathering information about the external environment, combining it with information received from the internal environment, and transmitting it to the higher centers of the brain including (but not limited to) the cerebellum, hypothalamus, thalamus, and cortex. When the information arrives at the cortex, incoming impulses are compared with information already stored. The sensory system transmits and processes information such as a pin prick, foot pressure, or joint position, from our external and internal environments. We have established that vertebrae are joints controlled by skeletal muscles, consequently, we can see that information from the muscles associated with the spine is transmitted in the same manner as is information concerning other joints.

Guyton also talks about another type of information — stored memory in the brain. Guyton is very specific (page 608 *The Sensory Division — Sensory Receptors*) about the staying-power of sensory input: "Most activities of the nervous system are originated by sensory experience emanating from *sensory receptors*, whether these be visual receptors, auditory receptors, tactile receptors on the surface of the body, or other kinds of receptors. This sensory experience can cause an immediate reaction, or its memory can be stored in the brain for minutes, weeks, or years and then can help to determine the bodily reactions at some future date."

The nervous system can draw upon and process past experiences that are stored in memory. In fact, Guyton's comment on page 609 (*Processing of Information*) is particularly significant: "More than 99 per cent of all sensory information is continually discarded by the brain as unimportant." Information such as tactile sensations generated by everyday stimuli such as the clothes we are wearing, most of the details of scenes within our field of vision, and continuous background noises are ignored. This concept is vital to an understanding of how and why chiropractic adjustments either work and last or merely move vertebrae temporarily, only to have them slip back to their pre-adjustment position as soon as the patient sits or stands. It becomes quite clear that our physiology, including vertebral position, is controlled largely by memory of past experiences.

Guyton's statement on page 610 (*Storage of Information — Memory*) is equally as significant to our understanding of the successful chiropractic adjustment. "Only a small fraction of the important sensory information causes an immediate motor response. Much of the remainder is stored for future control of motor activities and for use in the thinking processes. Most of this storage occurs in the *cerebral cortex*, but not all, for even the basal regions of the brain and perhaps even the spinal cord can store small amounts of information."

On the same page Guyton describes the role synapses play in determining the directions nerve signals take in traveling through the nervous system. He tells us: "The storage of information is the process we call *memory* and this too is a function of the synapses. That is, each time a particular sensory signal passes through a sequence of synapses, the respective synapses become more capable of transmitting the same signal the next time, which process is called *facilitation*. After the sensory signal has passed through the synapses a large number of times, the synapses become so facilitated that signals from the 'control center' of the brain can also cause transmission of impulses through the same sequence of synapses even though the sensory input has not been excited. This gives the person a perception of experiencing the original sensation, though in effect it is only a memory of the sensation." The particular sensory signals referred to can be generated by either external events or by internal stimuli such as memory of an event or a stressful situation. We can see by this how a patient's present physiology can be dramatically influenced by "re-runs" of past experiences.

On page 726, (*The Proprioceptor Feedback Servomechanism for Reproducing the Sensory Engram*), Guyton refers to cerebellar function and the role of proprioceptor signals in affecting motor activity. Proprioceptor signals also pass through the sensory areas of the cerebral cortex. "Once this pattern has been 'learned' by the sensory cortex, the memory engram of the pattern can be used to activate the motor system to perform the same sequential pattern whenever it is required." He then points out that the motor system acts as a servomechanism since the pattern for the activity is located in the sensory part of the brain and the motor system is following the pattern. "If ever the motor system fails to follow the pattern, sensory signals are fed back to the cerebral cortex to apprise the sensorium of this failure, and the appropriate corrective signals are transmitted to the muscles."

Guyton (page 726) illustrates the importance of sensory engrams in the control of motor movements by describing an experiment that involved removing parts of the cortex of monkeys that had been trained to perform some complex activities. "Removal of small portions of the motor cortex that control the muscles normally used for the activity does not prevent the monkey from performing the activity. Instead he automatically uses other muscles in place of the paralyzed ones to perform the same activity. On the other hand, if the corresponding somatic sensory cortex is removed but the motor cortex is left intact, the monkey loses *all* ability to perform the activity." This is a vivid illustration that input is more crucial to effecting a response than is output. This has a significant bearing on chiropractic in that we can see that the holding power of an adjustment is determined by the information going to the brain (input) rather than by the information coming from the brain (output).

The cortex and the thalamus, two of the "control centers" that Guyton referred to, are closely connected — afferent connections go from the thalamus to the cortex and efferent connections go from the cortex to the thalamus. All signals from four of the five senses — touch, sight, hearing, and taste — pass through the thalamus to the cortex and into either memory or conscious awareness; (the sense of smell is controlled by the hippocampus). The thalamus is aware of and responds to the conscious environment — we see it, hear it, touch it, taste it, and the thalamus knows about it. The hypothalamus, controls most of the involuntary functions of the body such as heart rate, blood pressure, body temperature and digestive functions. Internal stimuli from visceroceptors go to the hypothalamus which is responsible for homeostasis. Both the thalamus and hypothalamus, together with the cortex and cerebellum, play vital roles in how the body responds to chiropractic adjustment and to the *holding effect* of the adjustment.

On page 725, under the heading *Sensory Feedback Control of Motor Functions*, Guyton talks about "the relationship of the somatic sensory areas to the motor areas of the cortex" and "the close functional interdependence of the two areas." He goes on to say, "the somatic sensory area plays a major role in the control of motor functions"; and on page 710 (*Physiologic Anatomy of the Motor Areas of the Cortex and Their Pathways to the Cord*), "... the motor activities of the cortex are constantly controlled or modified by signals from the somatic sensory system." There is a sensory feedback mechanism involved in all motor function. This concept is illustrated by the Palmer "safety pin cycle." Guyton describes the physical intermingling of the areas of the precentral gyrus (motor) and postcentral gyrus (sensory): "Thus the two areas fade into each other with many somatic sensory fibers actually terminating directly in the motor cortex and some motor signals originating in the sensory cortex." It is significant to an analysis of the physiology of an adjustment to be aware that *motor signals originate in the sensory cortex* !

Guyton goes on to explain that "when a portion of the somatic sensory cortex in the postcentral gyrus is removed, the muscles controlled by the motor cortex immediately anterior to the removed area often lose much of the coordination." If an area of the sensory is removed, the motor function loses some of its ability. "This observation illustrates that the somatic sensory area plays a major role in the control of motor functions."

Guyton's observation also shows how important sensory impulses are to motor function. "The overall mechanism by which sensory feedback plays this role has been postulated to be the following: A person performs a motor movement mainly to achieve a purpose. It is primarily in the sensory and sensory association areas that he experiences effects of motor movements and records 'memories' of the different patterns of motor movements." This concept can be essential in understanding the effectiveness of vertebral adjustments. Every time a muscle moves, a memory of that movement is recorded in the sensory part of the central nervous system. "These are called sensory engrams of the motor movements." The pattern for this movement is recorded to be *replayed* in order to bring about that particular movement. "When he wishes to achieve some purposeful act, he presumably calls forth one of these engrams and then sets the motor system of the brain into action to reproduce the sensory pattern that is laid down in the engram."

SENSORY INFLUENCE ON MUSCLE ACTIVITY

There is no abnormal position of a vertebra that was not precipitated by a normal movement. Guyton speaks to this concept on page 685 (*Brain Areas for Control of the Gamma Efferent System*): "However, since the bulboreticular facilitatory area is particularly concerned with postural contractions, emphasis is given to the possible or probable important role of the gamma efferent mechanism in controlling muscle contraction for positioning the different parts of the body...." We can see by this statement that there is an area of the brain that is important in controlling the muscle contractions that position skeletal muscles and vertebrae.

All chiropractic adjustments by any technique are related to the sensory aspect of physiology. Although it may be thought that the effectiveness of an adjustment is due to altering motor function by relieving pressure through the IVF, it can be seen that any adjustment is in reality an indirect method of initiating a response from the motor system by updating the information that goes to the brain by the sensory system.

Mountcastle also emphasizes the role of the brain in controlling muscle activity (page 1771): "The cerebellum is a highly organized center that exerts a regulatory influence upon muscular activity. It receives a continuous stream of impulses relayed from receptors in muscles, joints, tendons, and skin and from visual, auditory and vestibular end organs. These impulses do not mediate conscious sensations, but they supply the sensory cues essential to the control of movement." Every action in the body is in response to at least one stimulus; there are no muscles designed to pull vertebrae out of position. Vertebrae may move out of position in response to particular stimuli, i.e., change of position, stress; however, if the vertebra stays in a position that fits a need no longer present, it is called a subluxation.

INTERCONNECTING INTERFERENCE, SUBLUXATIONS, AND DISEASE

Subluxation is seen by many as a direct cause of all disease. If, however, there is a direct relationship between the subluxation and disease, it is due to the position of the vertebrae which is dictating what is going *to* the central nervous system that, in turn, stimulates impulses coming *from* the brain through the IVF.

Interference, subluxations, and organ dysfunction are all interconnected; each element can either influence or be influenced by one or both of the other, as illustrated by this diagram.

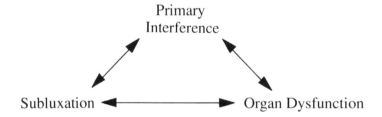

We have discussed how motor activity is a response to sensory signals stimulated by the position of the vertebrae. We understand that after a person twists to accomplish a normal function and the function is accomplished, the need to twist no longer exists; the memory is no longer appropriate and should be discarded after the action is complete. However, if the frequency or intensity of the impulse that precipitated the action was somehow altered in its ascent through the information system, the muscles and structure may receive the message to sustain the twisting position although this configuration is no longer necessary, and the person will experience stiffness, discomfort, pain, or subluxation.

Although the pain or sensations stem from structural misalignment, the source of the problem is in the memory engram patterns that stimulate the inappropriate structural response. Therefore, when a vertebra is adjusted, the release of pressure from the efferent nerves coming from the IVF is not the primary factor that influences the success of the adjustment. Releasing the pressure does have an impact; however, as we shall see in the discussion of muscle spindles, the impulses generated when a nerve is stimulated become both efferent and afferent. Mountcastle (page 1682) says that the reflex (contraction after stretching) action of a muscle "depended upon afferent signals from the muscle to the spinal cord, which elicited efferent responses returning to the muscle."

MUSCLE SPINDLES INFLUENCE VERTEBRAL POSITION

Chiropractic has concentrated on clearing the way for *efferent* signals to correct physiological dysfunction. When the study of physiology is correlated with an analysis of how chiropractic adjustments affect the totality of the body, we find that *afferent* signals exert the primary influence. It is clear that moving vertebrae is indeed an effective method of improving health. It is now becoming increasingly evident that removing interference at the IVF may not be the only goal of an adjustment. It is, in reality, a means of improving sensory input that will update memory patterns in order to achieve a more natural musculoskeletal response. The movement of vertebrae is a vehicle for accomplishing a lasting adjustment. This movement is more efficiently accomplished by updating memory patterns of the muscle spindles that control the length of muscles and Golgi tendon organs that control the tension of muscles. Unless the "memories" of these elements are updated, the adjustment will last only until the memory engram, via the righting reflex, reestablishes the former structural posture.

These principles apply to all techniques and the process occurs whether or not the chiropractor is aware that it is the sensorium that is being affected by manipulation. Manual application of force to move vertebrae, mechanical means of realigning the skeletal structure, or the application of subtle pressure can all convey information to the sensory aspect of the brain. The primary difference is whether the information is conveyed indirectly or directly to the sensory system. There is a greater margin for success in maintaining lasting adjustments with the direct approach — alerting the nervous system to the correct position — than there is in the indirect approach — manually altering the position of bones.

Sudden repositioning of bones can elicit the defense mechanism of the body (fight or flight reflex). It is this defensive reaction that may cause a compromise of the sensorial awareness that the vertebral position is inappropriate, thereby diluting the effectiveness of the adjustment. The direct approach (less force) does not elicit the body's natural defense reflexes which interfere with complete evaluation of the new muscle spindle tension.

Muscle memory is subcortical — subconscious. A patient cannot consciously relax a muscle if that muscle is being controlled by memory engram of a past experience transmitted through the subconscious. The memory that defines muscle length — determines whether the muscle will be relaxed or contracted — is a response to the stimulus that acts on the muscle spindle in conjunction with the Golgi tendon organ. Mountcastle explains the physiology of muscle spindles and Golgi tendon organs (page 1682): "Muscle spindles are located within the belly of the muscle. Because they are attached in parallel with other muscle fibers, they are stretched whenever the muscle is stretched. A receptor in each spindle responds to an increase of muscle length by generating action potentials at an increased rate. These receptors are therefore physiologic transducers that measure muscle length. Their signals are conducted to the spinal cord in type Ia nerve fibers, which involves a small but significant afferent delay...."

He continues (page 1698), "There is another type of stretch receptor in skeletal muscle, the Golgi tendon organ, which responds to an increase in tension rather than length. Tendon organs are located at the junctions of muscle fibers and their tendons, and thus they are in series with contractile parts of the muscle as opposed to the spindles, which are in parallel. They measure the forces produced by the contracting fibers and send impulses to the spinal cord by way of group Ib fibers. This afferent activity excites internuncial cells in the spinal cord, which in turn inhibit the motor neurons of the same muscle."

Guyton explains the importance of the role of muscle spindles and tendon organs in subconscious control of muscles (page 685, *Brain Areas for Control of the Gamma Efferent System*). "In addition to transmitting signals into the spinal cord, the muscle spindle also transmits signals up the cord to the cerebellum and thence into the bulboreticular areas.... However, both the signals that operate in the spinal cord and those that pass to the cerebellum are *entirely subconscious* [emphasis added], so that the conscious portion of the brain is never apprised of the immediate changes in length of the muscles." It is this subconscious memory pattern originating from the muscle spindles that, in a clinical setting, can account for the often observed situation of a patient's muscles continuing to remain tense and taut even after the tenseness has been noted and the patient has been asked to relax. Guyton continues: "On the other hand, ... signals from the joint receptors constantly apprise the conscious brain of the positions of the different parts of the body, even though the muscle receptors do not."

When a forceful adjustment is made, the lasting effects of that action relate indirectly to the muscle spindle, not directly to the new position of the joint. The muscle spindle picks up the new position, sends impulses up to the sensory areas of the brain, and if the signal comes back indicating that the new position has been established, the adjustment will hold. This sequence must take place every time in order for forceful adjustments to be successful. However, all that is actually necessary is for the muscle spindle information to be transmitted to the subconscious (to the bulbar area of the brain) so that the response transmitted through efferent fibers dictates a position that is more appropriate to the current situation. The muscles will then immediately relax and begin to work cooperatively, even if antagonistically, and will begin to reposition the vertebra appropriately to fit the need of the present situation.

DEFENSE RESPONSES

If we understand the association between the sensory and motor systems we see why forceful adjustments work on many occasions and why they do not work on other occasions. Chiropractic techniques have been effective partly because of the influence exerted directly on the muscle spindles by the brain.

It must be understood that any force applied to the body elicits some degree of defense response. This response may be manifest by tight muscles or tenseness such as occurs in the fight-or-flight reflex. When a sudden forceful adjustment causes a sudden change in the position of a vertebra, both rapid lengthening and rapid shortening of the attached antagonistic muscles will attempt to preserve the length. This reaction is, in effect, an attempt to maintain vertebral position that existed prior to the adjustment. Mountcastle addresses this (page 1683) when he says: "increases in muscle length that are produced by disturbing forces are sensed by spindle receptors which generate a larger feedback signal. As a result the motor neurons send a larger efferent nerve signal to the muscle (the controller), where the force of contraction is enhanced. The larger muscular force will counteract the disturbing force, tending to move the mass back toward its former position and the muscle toward its former length." Therefore, the reaction by the patient to an adjustment is diluted by the defense mechanism of the body in response to the force or trauma involved in the correction of a vertebral position.

Ideally, the body should be allowed to evaluate subconsciously, through the muscle spindles, the appropriateness of the vertebral position and to compare the findings with the appropriateness of a resting condition on the adjusting table. Only by providing updated information to establish new memory engrams which show that the reaction to a past traumatic experience is no longer appropriate will the body be able to maintain the new position of a suddenly altered position of vertebrae. Consequently, when the memory engrams are updated and the new position is accepted as appropriate, the muscles themselves will reposition the vertebrae and the need for manual repositioning no longer exists. By working through the sensory aspect of the central nervous system, chiropractic adjustments achieve the lasting health-producing effects that have served as the hallmark of the profession.

The body reacts exactly the same to all stress, real or imagined. A chiropractic approach that inflicts a degree of trauma (again either real or imagined) on the patient can often redefine the memory patterns to hold an adjustment. However, if a patient is at all anxious during an adjustment, whether the anxiety stems from conditions associated with his personal life or with the anticipation of the impending adjustment, the chances of this patient responding optimally are greatly decreased. Sensory information that is received is first evaluated in terms of stress — the need to adapt, or the fight-or-flight reflex. Hans Selye defines stress (page 64) as "the common denominator of all adaptive reactions in the body." Selye's work has identified the hypothalamus as the area of the central nervous system that initiates a response by the adrenal glands. On page 102 he describes "The role of the hypothalamus as a bridge between the brain and the endocrine system...." Clinical experience indicates that if the response pattern of the sensory signals that excite activity by the adrenals is stored in memory engrams, when this pattern is recalled for use, the adrenal response will be included. Each time this response pattern is stimulated, the adrenals will react. All stress is interpreted by the body as a real stress and the body's defense mechanisms react accordingly. This interpretation is an important element to be considered in the application of all procedures.

THE RIGHTING REFLEX

We have mentioned that the righting reflex can be activated when a patient sits or stands following an adjustment. This reflex can be seen as a function of the reticular formation, an area of the brain stem. Guyton (page 694, *The Reticular Formation, and Support of the Body Against Gravity*) locates the *reticular formation* as beginning at the upper end of the spinal cord and extending "(a) upward through the central portions of the thalamus, (b) into the hypothalamus, and (c) into other areas adjacent to the thalamus." Again, we can see that physiological responses are controlled by subconscious areas of the brain.

Guyton continues the description by giving the source of stimuli that go to the reticular formation. "The sensory input to the reticular formation is from multiple sources, including: (1) the spinoreticular tracts and collaterals from the spinothalamic tracts, (2) the vestibular tracts, (3) the cerebellum, (4) the basal ganglia, (5) the cerebral cortex, especially the motor regions, and (6) the hypothalamus and other nearby associated areas." We can see that these signals are from subconscious sources that can affect skeletal muscles. Since equilibrium and body position are controlled by subconscious memories, we can see that it is necessary for the memories to be updated if an adjustment is to hold after the patient sits or stands.

The righting reflex in a sitting position is different from that in a reclining position. Unless memory engrams have been updated during an adjustment, as soon as a patient sits up, all of memories for muscle spindle tension that are part of the righting reflex for the sitting position will come into play.

Every adjustment of every kind by any technique that is trying to influence a neurological change osseously involves competition. The competition is between the new position brought about by the adjustment, including how the patient responds, and memory of the righting reflex for an upright position that dictates a certain physiology. Chiropractic adjustments are aimed at causing a more appropriate response in the sitting position, and, in many instances, hoping for a more appropriate response in a standing stressless position.

Much is still to be learned about the workings of the human body as Mountcastle's statement (page 1775) shows: "Recordings from the surface of the cerebellum take the form of low-voltage sinusoidal waves recurring at rates of 100 to 300/sec. Superimposed on them is a continuous background of smaller fluctuations at frequencies of 1,000 to 2,000/sec. The origin of the latter type of activity is not established." As additional information is revealed through research, chiropractic will increase its knowledge base which will provide even more resources for helping patients.

We know from years of experience that there is a structure-function relationship that influences health. The body responds appropriately to each stimulus but osseous structures do not have the capacity for being judgmental. They cannot determine if they are in the position most advantageous to the patient's overall health. Bones, as all other entities of the body, are part of a systematic structure that is highly integrated — their positions are governed by stimuli affecting muscles and tendons. Bone is living tissue that responds to internal activity such as chemical reactions brought about by the food we eat, and to stress factors associated with life style. Bones respond to muscle action and their ultimate position is determined by lasting muscle tension.

SENSORY-MOTOR INTEGRATION — THE KEY TO LASTING ADJUSTMENTS

It is true that we have effected improved structure and improved health by chiropractic adjustments, and we have seen through scientific explanations how this occurs. Improved structure comes about not by the positioning and repositioning of the bones but by putting them in a more normal position that allows the muscle spindle to relax or tighten as appropriate. This, in turn, sends impulses to the sensory centers where memory engrams are established to maintain the improved position. Realizing the importance of sensory input to the condition and position of the skeletal system makes it possible to understand that the beneficial effects of all chiropractic adjustments, regardless of the technique used, have a lasting effect in that sensory-motor integration is improved. We can see that improved sensory-motor integration is the result of lasting chiropractic adjustment, and that lasting chiropractic adjustments depend on effecting improved sensory-motor integration.

The statements of Dr. Guyton and Dr. Mountcastle show that science has unwittingly already proved chiropractic if we will expand our concepts of what is involved in a chiropractic adjustment. Chiropractic can advance from merely citing clinical observations to a more firm scientific status by (1) associating scientific principles with our experience of improvements that have been brought about by moving vertebrae, and (2) assimilating the information gained from on-going research into our current storehouse of knowledge. In addition, our profession is open to relating to other scientific disciplines such as biochemistry and neurology that will foster an environment for other procedures that can benefit even more patients more consistently.

The work begun by the founders of our profession was the harbinger of a health care system that can provide healthful benefits to patients and satisfaction to chiropractors. However, in order to continue to improve our service to humanity, we must not only be constantly alert to advances in scientific knowledge but we must also be actively involved in uncovering additional information that will aid us in our growth and proficiency. Scientific research is not the exclusive domain of other scientific disciplines; chiropractic views the human body from a perspective different from that of most other health care systems, consequently, we are obligated to advance our scientific knowledge to the best of our abilities.

By expanding our concepts of chiropractic we can understand the underlying causes of why chiropractic adjustments do what we say they will do and we can realize even greater potential for greater good. We have accomplished amazing results for many patients without fully understanding exactly how the results came about. It is not absolutely necessary to know how something works for the process to be effective. Only a minute percentage of the world's population is aware that DNA is the key to genetic coding, yet this lack of information has not hindered reproduction of the species in the least. In the same vein, understanding exactly how the body responds to chiropractic adjustments is not absolutely essential to successfully treating patients, but a comprehensive view of how the body responds allows for greater understanding of what is taking place with each adjustment.

The future of chiropractic lies in acknowledging the role of the sensory system and working with the sensorium in order to effect the desired changes in the motor system. It is important for scientific researchers in physiology, neurology, anatomy and other disciplines, as well the highly skilled members of the chiropractic academic community to direct their attention to the integration of the sensory and motor systems. By correlating the sensory to the motor aspects of chiropractic we can extend our effectiveness in the healing arts. Our colleges of chiropractic are staffed by inquiring scientists who can lead the way in uncovering and disseminating the physiological reasons for our success to date. This knowledge will lead to a more comprehensive understanding of the physiology of the adjustment and to even greater success in the healing art of chiropractic in the future.

4

BIO ENERGETIC
SYNCHRONIZATION TECHNIQUE

THE EVOLUTION OF THE BIO ENERGETIC
SYNCHRONIZATION TECHNIQUE

Bio Energetic Synchronization Technique is a system of chiropractic care that has evolved over the past seventeen years in response to my perception of the need for procedures that will consistently effect positive spinal structural improvement.

Bio Energetic Synchronization is an outgrowth of extensive experience with other chiropractic techniques including Logan Basic, Gonstead, Diversified, and Kinesiology which were used in my practice for several years. While the results achieved with these procedures were gratifying, I determined that positive results should be not only the rule but should be attained without exception.

The development of the Bio Energetic Synchronization Technique has been evolving since 1974 in an effort to meet the needs of my patients. Although the application of the technique undergoes modifications and refinements as additional information becomes available, the basic premises have remained unchanged. In an article published in the January/February 1976 edition of *The Digest of Chiropractic Economics*, I wrote of the important role stress plays in determining health, "... we assumed that all pain was caused by physical trauma. In reality, the cause may well have been from an emotional trauma or mental taxation, and only the effect is physical." Also in this issue, as in other articles, I asked for comments and criticisms concerning my views and findings.

In the November/December 1976 issue, I was concerned with the intricate communication between the internal and external environments: "Our external environment and our internal environment must be in constant communication and they must reflect and interact continuously. Each of these reactions will have an effect on the total distribution of the body's energy. In health, all of these shifts and compensations are made automatically without our even being aware of them."

I was aware that most chiropractors thought of themselves as motor doctors affecting only that part of the central nervous system. In the January/February 1981 issue of *The American Chiropractor*, I encouraged expansion of our concepts to consider the roles the sensory system and previous experiences play in sustaining vertebral corrections: "If you reposition that vertebra and the brain is not made aware of it, then the brain will reposition that vertebra exactly where it was before you made the move. It has to. The brain was aware of its malposition in the first place. The brain was aware by way of proprioceptors that give us information on muscle equilibrium, and the position and tension of joints!!"

The Bio Energetic Synchronization Technique has led me toward my goal of an increased rate of successful adjustments. As is frequently the case in any developmental process, an unexpected series of events served as a catalyst. Events in my personal and professional lives were closely interwoven in a way that led me to recognize a different perspective as to how the body reacts to vertebrae being moved. Subsequently, initial investigations served as the foundation for relating physiological responses to adjustments and also for the realization that by augmenting existing methodology, I could increase my level of successful patient responses.

During all of the investigations, the principles and goals of chiropractic have remained intact:

- chiropractic treats the whole person rather than merely symptoms,

- chiropractic recognizes a structure-function relationship that influences total health,

- chiropractic is a method of health care administered by use of the hands on the spine and related areas,

- chiropractic removes obstructions that impede the flow of nerve impulses,

- chiropractic is a drugless, non-surgical alternative health care discipline,

- chiropractic recognizes that the power that made the body can heal the body, and

- chiropractic treats the cause, not the effect, of disease.

With these principles as a basis, Bio Energetic Synchronization Technique methods allow the body (1) to provide the action that adjusts vertebrae, (2) to synchronize the many physiological systems of the body, and (3) to update the memory patterns that evoke responses to sensory stimuli.

The impact of any chiropractic adjustment is extensive — each adjustment affects the entire body rather than only the local area involved. A deeper understanding of the physiology of both subluxations and adjustments has been gained from recent research leading to the correlation and interpretation of the extent of the influence an adjustment has on the body. It is no longer necessary for chiropractic to stand in the shadows of quasi-scientific explanations. Chiropractic has long offered and fulfilled the promise of health-restoring aid to those in physical distress. By applying accepted physiological concepts, it is possible to relate the means of chiropractic adjustments to the end results.

As chiropractors, we are ultimately concerned with vertebral position. We have addressed the physiology of an adjustment, what happens when a vertebra is adjusted, and have shown that the lower levels of the brain act as the control center for vertebral position. Bio Energetic Synchronization Technique provides a direct communication with this control center.

The Bio Energetic Synchronization Technique is predicated on the principle that the body always responds correctly to the stimuli it receives. If the response is such that the patient is in a degree of distress, relief can be achieved by changing the stimulus that caused the distress. This principle can be applied to a variety of common responses such as headaches, diabetes, osteoporosis, rheumatoid diseases, high blood pressure, and, of course, inappropriate structural alignment, to name just a few. No claims are made that the Bio Energetic Synchronization Technique will cure any disease, nor is this health care system presented as a treatment for disease. The only curative power in existence resides within the body. This technique does allow the body to become totally aware of the actual condition of the body.

STIMULUS AND RESPONSE

In order to alter negative responses — which are perfectly attuned to the stimulus or stimuli that precipitated them — the stimulus must be changed to one that will elicit a more positive response. Treating the response (crisis therapy) may bring temporary relief, but for lasting improvement in health, the stimulus, or cause, must be determined and addressed.

An axiom of Bio Energetic Synchronization Technique is "The body doesn't know how to be sick." The body is primarily a response mechanism that, in its own right, does not have one system, organ, fiber or cell that is designed to initiate or prolong illness. Everything in the body is geared toward perfect health; every response in the body is to a specific stimulus, and the stimulus may be either external or internal, of short duration or of long duration, intense or subtle. Detecting and recognizing the particular stimulus that elicits a particular response is the role of the doctor regardless of the technique used.

Despite the many forms that negative responses can take (as illustrated by the vast array of disease names used by the medical community to identify specific negative response patterns), only three underlying factors precipitate stimuli which will express negative responses. These factors are classified in general terms as "toxicity," "timing," and "thoughts."

"Toxicity," or autointoxication, is essentially due to forcing the body to adapt its physiology in order to metabolize and eliminate inappropriate foods or excesses of foods in an effort to achieve homeostasis. Toxicity ordinarily is built up over a long period of time by adhering to diets that may be culturally correct but are physiologically disastrous.

Interference brought about by impaired communication within the individual is a "timing" problem; the body is responding in precisely the correct manner for a situation that may no longer exist. Every part of the body is supposed to be synchronized with every other part of the body at all times. If the body's timing is not synchronized, discomfort or organ dysfunction is manifest. Chiropractic has historically addressed inappropriate timing through vertebral adjustments — when a chiropractic adjustment is successful, the body's timing has been synchronized. Our experience shows that timing problems occur when present physiology is being dictated by past experiences that are stored in memory.

The third cause of disease is "thoughts." We know that a well-nourished, well-timed body can become ill through habitually negative thoughts. We have seen that any stimulus, real or imagined, elicits a response by the body, and thoughts are equally as potent stimuli as concrete experiences.

COMMUNICATING WITH THE SENSORY SYSTEM

The Bio Energetic Synchronization Technique can be described as a direct approach in communicating with the sensory system to consistently bring about results that are frequently brought about indirectly by other chiropractic techniques. It is a form of holistic health care that integrates the many systems of the body by addressing nerve imbalances in sensory-motor functions to correct a primary interference that can be the root cause of organ dysfunction or pain, including what is commonly referred to as subluxation.

It is an underlying premise of the Bio Energetic Synchronization Technique that greater patient benefit can be derived by working with the sensory system without eliciting the defense mechanism that comes of using force.

The Bio Energetic Synchronization Technique allows the doctor to speak to each of these interference situations through the sensory system of the patient in order to coordinate cortical and subcortical control over muscles to bring about improved *vertebral position*. We employ body language, which is a motor response, and this technique communicates with the body through vestibular, respiration, vision, somesthetic, and kinesthetic methods of communication.

As the Bio Energetic Synchronization Technique system of chiropractic care has grown, academic research into accepted scientific texts has clarified clinical results and supported our scientific precepts. Founded on the chiropractic principles taught in our accredited colleges, only the perspective concerning the sensory-motor relationship has been expanded to facilitate a scientifically verifiable system of chiropractic.

The Bio Energetic Synchronization Technique system utilizes leg length (a traditional chiropractic evaluative procedure), arm strength, and vertebral position and tenderness as the standards to determine the physiological balance of each patient.

Bio Energetic Synchronization Technique offers methods of searching for, identifying, and removing interferences that foster an environment in which subluxations can occur or be retained. The basic clinical technique of Bio Energetic Synchronization centers around pressure applied by hand to strategic points on the spine as well as other areas of the body. These points are revealed through palpation of the tender and/or spastic areas of the body that are indicated, by response to testing for variations in leg length, to be priority centers of nerve interference. The subtle yet precise pressure that is applied disperses blocked nerve energy, eliminates physiological interference that segments the body, paves the way for more balanced input of sensory signals to all levels of the central nervous system, and allows improvement in both vascular circulation and nerve impulse flow that mandates improved vertebral position.

For a new vertebral position to be maintained after force has been applied to achieve that position, the *reaction* of the body to the new position is more important than the new position itself. Specific adjustments of the vertebral articulations will release fixations and stimulate sensory fibers to carry impulses to the brain for evaluation. If the adjusted position is more correct for present conditions than the pre-adjustment position, the motor response will attempt to maintain the improved position. However, if the newly corrected vertebral position is not accepted by the controlling, integrating area of the brain (memory engram), the paravertebral muscles will again receive the compensated impulses that allowed the subluxation to occur initially. As soon as the patient sits up and re-engages the righting reflex, gravity will again force the vertebra into a less than perfect position (subluxation).

COMMUNICATION WITHIN THE BODY

Bio Energetic Synchronization operates on the premise that the afferent (sensory) nerves going into the intervertebral foramen become primarily responsible for maintaining a newly corrected vertebral position.

We have seen that manual repositioning of vertebrae may indirectly bring about a lasting change in vertebral position. Guyton shows that joint position (vertebral position) is determined by the information sent by the muscle spindles and the Golgi tendon apparatus to the cerebellum, and Mountcastle points out (page 1715): "The main function of the three types of receptors in muscle is in the subconscious control of muscles." The Bio Energetic Synchronization system, working with these physiological conditions, has a direct effect on vertebral position through the sensory system.

Guyton addresses a very important concept of Bio Energetic Synchronization Technique in his discussion of proprioceptive feedback and sensory engrams. Recall that "proprioception" refers to the appraisal by the body of the position of all muscles and joints. Guyton states (page 726, *The Proprioceptor Feedback Servomechanism for Reproducing the Sensory Engram*), "From the earlier discussion of cerebellar function, it is clear how proprioceptor signals from the periphery can affect motor activity." Part of the lengthy discussion to which Guyton refers concerns the extreme importance of the cerebellum's activities although the cerebellum has no *direct* control over muscle contraction. He states on page 717 (*The Cerebellum and its Motor Functions*), "... it makes corrective adjustments in the motor activities elicited by other parts of the brain. It receives continuously updated information from the peripheral parts of the body to determine the instantaneous status of each part of the body — its position, its rate of movement, forces acting on it, and so forth. The cerebellum *compares* the actual physical status of each part of the body as depicted by the sensory information with the status that is intended by the motor system. If the two do not compare favorably, then appropriate corrective signals are transmitted instantaneously back into the motor system to increase or decrease the levels of activation of the specific muscles."

One important reason that the body does not innately or automatically correct subluxation is that all vertebral positions were correct for some past need, therefore, the positions are not recognized as a threat to homeostasis. It has been postulated that any physical condition of the body is created or tolerated by the brain, including the memory engrams that Guyton so adequately addresses.

Mountcastle's opening description of the cerebellum (page 1771) that emphasizes the importance of the role it plays in muscular activity is particularly significant to procedures incorporated in the Bio Energetic Synchronization Technique. "The cerebellum is a highly organized center that exerts a regulatory influence upon muscular activity. It receives a continuous stream of impulses relayed from receptors in muscles, joints, tendons, and skin and from visual, auditory, and vestibular end organs. These impulses do not mediate conscious sensations, but they supply the sensory cues essential to the control of movement. Signals from the cerebral cortex and other motor regions also reach the cerebellar nuclei. Some of this influx terminates in the cerebellar nuclei, but most of it is distributed through an elaborate network to the Purkinje cells of the cortex."

Mountcastle goes on to say: "The nuclear cells are thus subject to the effects of afferent impulses which reach them directly and to the integrated outflow of the cortex. From the nuclei, fibers pass to the thalamus, red nucleus, vestibular nuclei, and reticular formation of the brain stem. Through these connections the cerebellum influences motor centers from the cerebral cortex to the spinal motor neurons, modifying the control of muscular action from the level of its inception to that of its execution."

DIRECT COMMUNICATION

An objective of the Bio Energetic Synchronization Technique adjustment is to allow the cerebellum and all of the subcortical areas of the brain to directly receive accurate updated information concerning present conditions including the position of the vertebrae. This information is essential in order for the responses to be appropriate to current need rather than to the myriad of compensations previously used through memory engram control that elicited responses to circumstances no longer present.

To communicate directly with subcortical levels of the central nervous system, five body languages are used in the Bio Energetic Synchronization Technique: vestibular, vision, respiration, kinesthetic, and somesthetic. Each of these is very specific and relates to a particular level of the central nervous system. The languages all represent very precise sensory input that initiates motor responses providing information appropriate for the current resting physiology of the patient.

Using the five body languages allows updated information to be transmitted into that part of the brain that is responsible for maintaining vertebral position. This is the direct way to accomplish a lasting correction. Any, and perhaps all, of these five body languages can be influenced by a conventional vertebral adjustment, but it is usually through indirect communication.

In the Bio Energetic Synchronization Technique, the five languages are used both as an assessment device and as a therapeutic medium. An overview of the methods of communicating with the body through the five languages will be helpful in understanding how Bio Energetic Synchronization stimulates the vertebral repositioning that can lead to an improvement in overall physiology.

The adjustment is given with the patient lying relaxed on the table, and, ideally, with the anti-gravity proprioceptor muscles in a relaxed state. However, the proprioceptive muscles are controlled 99% by memory engrams, and many of these engrams may, without the patient realizing it, still be responding to a crisis situation which demanded that a particular muscle be tight. When the body is allowed to update these engrams through direct communication with the higher levels of the nervous system, the tight muscles will relax and vertebrae will be allowed to resume their correct position. Physiological communication through one or a combination of these languages has consistently resulted in improved leg-length and/or arm-strength parity.

VESTIBULAR COMMUNICATION

In a Bio Energetic Synchronization adjustment the patient assumes a recumbent position and resting physiology, and the doctor checks the evenness of leg length. None of the postural muscles should be active in this position. On request of the doctor, the patient turns his head which immediately initiates a new vestibular response. The leg lengths are again compared. An alteration in leg lengths as a result of turning the head indicates that an area of interference at a high brain level is involved. Guyton shows this connection on page 698 (*Neuronal Connections of the Vestibular Apparatus with the Central Nervous System*) when he cites the origin of the reflexes for equilibrium: "The primary pathway for the reflexes of equilibrium begins in the vestibular nerves and passes next to both the vestibular nuclei and the cerebellum. Then, after much two-way traffic of impulses between these two, signals are sent into the reticular nuclei of the brain stem as well as down the spinal cord via the vestibulospinal and reticulospinal tracts."

Early in the development of this technique, it was observed that the position of the patient's head also had an effect on muscle strength. The body is very much concerned with the position of the head in relation to the position of the rest of the body and is equipped with several mechanisms to monitor and evaluate this information. Guyton elaborates on this (page 696, *Support of the Body Against Gravity*): "When a person or an animal is in a standing position, continuous impulses are transmitted from the reticular formation and from closely allied nuclei, particularly from the vestibular nuclei, into the spinal cord and thence to the extensor muscles to stiffen the limbs. This allows the limbs to support the body against gravity. These impulses are transmitted mainly by way of the reticulospinal and vestibulospinal tracts." If the postural muscles remain in a contracted state while the patient is relaxed on the table, it is obvious that the contraction is in response to the memory of standing and is no longer appropriate.

The vestibular apparatus is located in the inner ear. The cochlear duct is concerned with hearing and has nothing to do with vestibular, however, the utricle, the saccule, and the semi-circular canals are especially important in maintaining equilibrium as they apprise the sensorium of the position of the head. "Most of the vestibular fibers end in the vestibular nuclei, which are located approximately at the junction of the medulla and the pons, but some fibers pass without synapsing to the fastigial nuclei, uvula, and flocculonodular lobes of the cerebellum" (Guyton page 697, *Neuronal Connections of the Vestibular Apparatus with the Central Nervous System*). When the body provides the doctor with a negative response (such as a "weak arm" when the head is turned) this is an indication of nerve interference at this level of the central nervous system. Conversely, a positive response (a "strong arm") indicates a lack of interference. The Bio Energetic Synchronization adjustment, in the correction of a vestibular problem, removes interference above the spinal segments. As long as the interference remains, the negative response will be evident 100% of the time.

In the section "Function of the Utricle and the Saccule in the Maintenance of Static Equilibrium" (page 698), Guyton talks about the nervous system being apprised of "the position of the head with respect to the pull of gravity. In turn, the vestibular, cerebellar, and reticular motor systems reflexly excite the appropriate muscles to maintain proper equilibrium."

If we make a vertebral adjustment without updating the memory engrams associated with vestibular and the righting reflex, then as soon as the patient stands up, the engrams again become dominant and force the same compensations upon all postural muscles as well as spinal muscles. Joseph G. Chusid, M.D., and Joseph J. McDonald, M.D., in their textbook, *Correlative Neuroanatomy and Functional Neurology*, (Lange

Medical Publications, Los Altos, California, 1962, p. 44), tell us there are five righting reflexes. "The righting reflexes function to maintain the top side uppermost: (1) Labyrinthine righting reflexes maintain the head's orientation in space and require an intact midbrain. (2) Body righting reflexes acting upon the head keep the head orientated with respect to the body and require an intact midbrain. (3) Body righting reflexes acting upon the body, arising from receptors on the body surfaces, tend to keep the body orientated in space and require an intact midbrain. (4) Neck righting reflexes arising in the neck keep the body orientated with respect to the head and require an intact medulla. (5) Optical righting reflexes keep the head in proper orientation and depend upon an intact occipital cortex."

Any one or several of these reflexes may be compensated by a trauma-imprinted memory engram. A Bio Energetic Synchronization Technique adjustment removes interference from all of these neurological areas without engaging any of the five righting reflexes. This gives an integrated total body response by utilizing selective individual sensory input to each area to update the "error" in the memory engram. Each area is cleared while the patient is lying on the adjusting table and the righting reflexes are inactive. When the patient stands, a new, uncompensated engram is imprinted which provides physiology more appropriate to present need or intent.

In explaining how a difference or "error" in memory engrams can be corrected, on page 726 (*The Proprioceptor Feedback Servomechanism for Reproducing the Sensory Engram*) Guyton tells us, "If ever the motor system fails to follow the pattern, sensory signals are fed back to the cerebral cortex to apprise the sensorium of this failure, and appropriate corrective signals are transmitted to the muscles." Bio Energetic Synchronization communicates directly with these high brain centers through light force applied to the spine and related areas, thereby allowing the update to occur and permitting a new, more nearly normal engram to be formed.

All of the procedures incorporated in the Bio Energetic Synchronization Technique are methods of analysis to search for weakness (primarily exhibited in the extremities) which indicates that interference exists in an area of the central nervous system. This technique utilizes tests of arm strength as an indicator of nerve interference in the lower areas of the brain.

With the patient supine on the adjusting table, one arm at a time is raised and the patient rotates or laterally flexes the head. If interference exists, rotating the head to one side weakens resistance to slight pressure on an upraised arm; however, it might be necessary to laterally flex the head, or include rotation along with lateral flexion. It becomes evident that muscle weakness caused by changing the position of the head indicates that interference in nerve impulse flow exists and that motor signals from other parts of the body are involved and influenced. Investigation has confirmed the relationship between arm strength and changes in head position. The rotation or flexion of the cervical spine preparatory to any adjustment immediately puts a new vestibular impulse into the subconscious. Therefore, merely specific rotation of the neck can transmit information that can update engrams and have a therapeutic effect.

VISION COMMUNICATION

Vision is probably the single most important factor in sensory input. In addition to the faculty of seeing, vision is important in vestibular as well as other functions, especially the visual righting reflex. Visual impulses pass from the retina to the lateral geniculate body which lies in close proximity to the optic tract and the optic radiations. From the geniculate body, impulses travel to the visual cortex; however, many fibers carrying visual information also go to the cerebellum indicating that this information will be used in a subconscious function.

Since patients ordinarily spend most of their waking time in an upright position with their eyes open, the engrams for upright posture and eyes-open become very closely associated. Mountcastle tells us on page 1695, "Maintenance of upright posture and balance requires vestibular feedback. A large part of all voluntary motor activity is guided by visual feedback." When the patient lies down, he ordinarily has his eyes closed and another set of engrams controls this position. In a Bio Energetic Synchronization Technique adjustment, the patient opens his eyes for a given series of sensory input activities then closes his eyes for other sensory input activities. This makes it possible to determine whether or not resting physiology is compensated by upright memory postural engrams.

Patients will exhibit a definite difference in ability to resist lightly applied pressure when the arms are tested for resistance strength to compare responses between eyes-open with eyes-closed. Again, the weakness indicates that there is interference at some point along the visual pathway. All of the visual pathways that are involved are deep in the central nervous system and close to the most vital areas of the brain. Any type of adjustment given while the patient is prone will accomplish sensory input whether or not the eyes are open since the visual apparatus is inactive in this position.

Removal of all interference in the correlation and interpretation of visual signals from the higher levels of the brain is necessary for complete correction as the visual centers are closely associated with the righting reflex. Finding negative indications after the patient sits up shows that former compensatory engrams associated with the righting reflex engrams have overridden the adjustment, and, similarly, a sustained adjustment indicates that the interference has been removed.

RESPIRATION COMMUNICATION

Guyton indicates that there is no precise respiratory center in the central nervous system; however, neurogenic mechanisms in the medulla and pons can provide almost complete respiration stimulation even when higher centers have been destroyed. Therefore, this area of the brain stem is referred to as the respiratory center. Interference at this level is manifest by a marked difference in muscle strength of the arms between inspiration and exhalation, and an equalization of strength between the two states, taken along with positive clinical findings, indicates a removal of the interference. As with other analysis techniques, it is the difference in muscle strength under opposing conditions (exhalation and inhalation) that is significant.

Generally, we are inclined to think of homeostasis as the regulation of the internal functions of the body and, of course, this is correct as far as it goes. However, structure is also a function of homeostasis. The maintenance of correct muscle tone and all the proprioceptive impulses are under the umbrella of homeostasis which is controlled subconsciously by the hypothalamus. The respiratory centers of the brain function at a subcortical level and are also monitored by the hypothalamus. Guyton tell us (page 557, Chapter 42, *Regulation of Respiration*), "The nervous system adjusts the rate of alveolar ventilation almost exactly to the demands of the body...." Any compensations resulting from past experiences that affect respiration could affect posture and muscle strength. Guyton includes erector spinal muscles in a list of muscles of inspiration (page 517, *The Muscles of Inspiration and Expiration*). Consequently, any tightness or spasm of the spinal muscles associated with subluxation could affect respiration.

Perhaps the greatest amount of influence exerted on respiration by the subconscious is by way of emotions. When a person is immersed in very cold water, he immediately, and involuntarily, gasps — sudden inspiration. Gasping is a response that can be associated with sudden trauma or stress; consequently, respiration associated with anxiety can be recorded in a memory engram along with defensive muscle responses. This composite of anxiety-produced responses could be referred to as a trauma engram.

Most trauma engrams are imprinted during some phase of the inspiration-exhalation cycle while the person is in an upright position. The trauma engram can be imprinted with the amount of respiration present at the time of the event which can cause compensation of all future respiration.

We know from experience that many emotional states can affect the character of respiration — fear, anxiety, rage, and other high intensity emotions. When we recall that 99% of sensory information is discarded, it can be seen how a traumatic memory engram associated with a strong emotion could significantly alter respiration. For most patients, some degree of adrenal stress response accompanied a situation that led to a subluxation or organ dysfunction. This adrenal response should be considered in the correction.

Since most adjustments are given with the patient lying down, it is significant to recall that pulmonary volumes and capacities are affected by posture. In the section entitled *Significance of the Pulmonary Volumes and Capacities*, (page 522), Guyton states, "... the different 'volumes' and 'capacities' change with the position of the body, most of them decreasing when the person lies down and increasing when he stands." Most chiropractors instruct the patient to exhale just prior to the thrust. Although the physiological justification for exhalation at this time may not be recognized, clinical experience has shown it to be helpful.

KINESTHETIC COMMUNICATION

According to Guyton (page 651, *Kinesthetic Sensations*), "The term 'kinesthesia' means conscious recognition of the orientation of the different parts of the body with respect to each other as well as of the rates of movement of the different parts of the body. These functions are subserved principally by extensive sensory endings in the joint capsules and ligaments."

Bio Energetic Synchronization procedures not only search for weakness but also seek to correct inappropriate engram patterns. This can be accomplished by kinesthetic communication through the conscious turning and flexing of the feet by the patient in a supine position, again utilizing the eyes-open and eyes-closed technique. Repetitive movements of the feet generate impulses through the muscle spindles and Golgi tendon apparatus to indicate a more normal range of motion. This method of consciously affecting the subconscious through repetitive actions allows engrams to be updated to be more appropriate to present need.

By having the patient turn his feet in and out as a part of a precise series of sensory input activities, a change in arm muscle strength can be observed. This in turn indicates changes in the kinesthetic areas of the brain. Conscious thought is required for the patient to turn his feet in and out. This activity provides a conscious stimulus which is carried by the muscle spindles. The revised stimulus can then be compared to the pattern already held in the subconscious regardless of whether the original pattern was formed from sensory input or from memory. This allows for more complete integration of conscious and subconscious actions. Again, communication is directly established with the area of the brain that is ultimately responsible for vertebral position.

A part of a Bio Energetic Synchronization adjustment may involve the passive movement of various parts of the body. For example, with the patient prone and knees flexed at a 45° angle, if the patient is relaxed, the legs should fall to the table when support is withdrawn. However, if they remain at the same angle although the patient believes he is relaxed, this indicates that his physiology is being controlled by memory engrams. To restructure the engrams that are causing the legs to remain flexed, a more favorable resting posture and updated engram pattern can be established by the legs being moved passively through a range of motion while applying pressure to the belly of the muscle (in this case the hamstring). This puts an updated proprioceptive signal into the muscle spindle. This signal goes to the subconscious which will recognize that the movement is indeed passive and that it is no longer necessary to respond as if the hamstring were defying gravity. The subconscious will update its activity and allow the hamstring to relax. Once this is achieved, we know that we have communicated with an area of the brain that is responsible for joint position and muscle tension which, as we have established, includes vertebral position.

SOMESTHETIC COMMUNICATION

The Bio Energetic Synchronization Technique utilizes physiological concepts pertaining to the tactile transmission of information in somesthetic communication to directly affect sensory-motor interference problems through specific contacts on various parts of the body. In a Bio Energetic Synchronization Technique adjustment, very precise contacts are taken on areas of the spine. These may be on the spinous process, on a transverse process, or, often, on the lateral areas of the posterior surface of the sacrum. In addition to these spinal points, contacts are made on the head. Cephalic contacts, also very specific, are used to directly affect the sensory and motor areas of the cortex to facilitate removal of interference at this level. Areas of subluxation and fixations are located and adjusted allowing the paravertebral muscles to assume more normal positions since updated information is able to reach them.

Guyton explains the path of information from one part of the nervous system to another on page 632 (*Transmission of Spatial Patterns Through Successive Neuronal Pools*): "... sensory information from the skin passes first through the peripheral nerve fibers, then through second order neurons that originate either in the spinal cord or in the cuneate and gracile nuclei of the medulla, and finally through third order neurons originating in the thalamus to the cerebral cortex."

We know that dermatomes throughout the body are associated with certain spinal levels and that just touching the skin initiates muscle spindle activity. These dermatomes are also associated with referred pain and thereby influence internal organ physiology.

Mountcastle also addresses cutaneous responses on page 1740: "The sensory receptors in skin and subcutaneous tissues respond to touch, pressure, heat, cold, and tissue damage. The signals from all of these receptors exert reflex effects on spinal motor neurons via internuncial cells." Mountcastle describes how afferent fibers from the skin transmit to the internuncial cells in the dorsal horn, and he goes on to say, "The responses of motor neurons are frequently very similar to those of certain interneurons in their time course, which indicates that the patterning of motor responses may be quite a direct consequence of internuncial activity."

Clinical experience has demonstrated that extremely light finger pressure applied to the body can provide direct communication with the central nervous system. The evaluation technique used to determine weakness indicates the areas of the body (other than the area of chief complaint) where points of tenderness will be found. Generally, until palpation, the patient is unaware that these tender areas exist. Specific tender points, characterized by small soft edematous, or hard pea-like nodules, that can be detected by palpation are commonly found right over the spinous or transverse processes. Doctors trained in the Bio Energetic Synchronization Technique are able to detect subtle yet distinct pulses by applying sustained gentle pressure to these nodules.

Anatomical pulses are phenomena in human physiology that are worthy of additional research by the scientific community. Pulses are present in all stages of human existence beginning before the union of egg and sperm. We know that the egg and sperm pulsate separately and independently, yet the moment they unite, only one pulse is present. As the fertilized ovum divides, the newly formed daughter cells pulsate in synchronization. This phenomenon has been demonstrated by photomicrographs.

David J. Meletich and Associates reported in *Toxicology and Applied Pharmacology* 70, 1983, that rat heart cells placed in a petri dish would all achieve a synchronized pulse after three or four days. The fact that embryonic cells pulsate in harmony implies that all cells should pulsate in synchronization. However, although our clinical observations and research have shown that pulses throughout the body are not always in harmony, by applying gentle pressure to two equally tender areas of the body, within a matter of seconds, the pulses will usually synchronize. Synchronized pulsations on the contact points in conjunction with the five body languages indicate that interference at the high brain levels has been removed. Holding these pulses to verify synchronization signifies improved body symmetry that is evidenced consistently by equal leg lengths.

It is through these light-pressure adjustments that the memory engrams are updated to allow the body to recognize more appropriate structural configuration. In addition, as with all chiropractic techniques, improved structural position can positively influence organ function. Organ function responds to the chiropractic adjustment in exactly the same way as does structural improvement. Muscle spindles are affected by the adjustment and impulses are transmitted to the cerebellum which, in turn, responds by transmitting efferent impulses which initiate motor response.

Frequently, auxiliary contacts are taken on the abdomen during a Bio Energetic Synchronization adjustment. H.B. Logan suggested as early as 1935 that abdominal contact is very important in the Basic technique. Abdominal contacts have a dual effect. First, they allow relaxation of the muscle spindles of the abdominal muscles which are tight in response to the defensive stress reaction; and second, these contacts have an effect on the visceral afferent. Guyton states in the seventh edition of his physiology textbook (1986), that "80 per cent of the nerve fibers in the vagus nerve are afferent rather than efferent" (page 757). Since the vagus nerve is 20% motor and 80% sensory, we can see that when the vagus is affected, impulses are transmitted to the hypothalamus. We have established that impulses that reach the hypothalamus can affect homeostasis including visceral function. Although neither relaxing the abdominal muscles nor the effect on visceral function is dependent upon the other, they occur at the same time which explains the concept of the triangulation of primary interference, subluxation, and organ dysfunction. Interference at high brain levels can cause both subluxation and organic malfunction.

Abdominal contacts taken in conjunction with contacts on the spine bring about communication between the sympathetic and parasympathetic nervous systems through the sacrum and spine. Inappropriate memory engrams that control visceral function can be updated to allow natural homeostatic correction of organ function just as corrected vertebral position is brought about by updated musculoskeletal patterns. For instance, if the stomach continues to respond to a stress that is no longer present, improved communication and updating of memory engrams can allow the body's natural homeostasis-seeking tendencies to improve gastric function to be more appropriate for present non-stress need.

Guyton describes the close relationship between the viscera and specific dermatomes resulting from the origin of the embryonic organs. (*Localization of Referred Pain Transmitted by the Visceral Pathways*, page 670): "Because the visceral afferent pain fibers are responsible for transmitting referred pain from the viscera, the location of the referred pain on the surface of the body is in the dermatome of the segment from which the visceral organ was originally derived in the embryo." Abdominal and spinal contacts can be effective for patients who suffer from referred pain.

CONSISTENT CHIROPRACTIC CORRECTIONS

Proper application of Bio Energetic Synchronization Technique procedures by a trained practitioner utilizing these five languages will *always* accomplish chiropractic corrections. These procedures can and have been effective for patients of all ages from newborns to nineties. Since the system is completely nonforceful, it is well-suited to children, the elderly, those in severe pain, and pregnant women.

Using the Bio Energetic Synchronization Technique, objectively verifiable structural realignment along with subjectively observed symptomatic improvement is the rule.

Included in the Appendix are representative examples of before and after x-rays and laboratory analysis data that illustrate the results obtained consistently through the application of Bio Energetic Synchronization Technique procedures.

5

SUMMARY

This paper has reviewed the unique position chiropractic holds in the health care field, offered a view based on accepted scientific principles of the impact of chiropractic adjustments on the many anatomical and physiological systems of the body, and presented an overview of the Bio Energetic Synchronization Technique as a chiropractic procedure that utilizes chiropractic and scientific principles to directly address the source of interference.

The three fundamental concepts on which the Bio Energetic Synchronization Technique focus are:

1. interference must be removed at high-brain levels by updating response patterns to sensory stimuli or memory engrams;

2. sensory input has a greater effect on motor response than has been previously acknowledged; and,

3. approximately 99% of a person's present physiology is controlled by responses to past experiences.

Clinical experience with the Bio Energetic Synchronization Technique has demonstrated consistent positive results by patients as substantiated by:

1. pre-treatment and post-treatment x-rays showing marked improvement in structure;

2. blood profiles and x-rays showing improvement in physiological function; and,

3. patients' assessments of symptom improvement as reflected by comments relative to comfort level.

6

CONCLUSIONS

Traditional core chiropractic has experienced significant success for almost 100 years by focusing on the influence vertebral position has on musculoskeletal integrity and somatic function. Clinical experience in conjunction with scientific investigation has led to a more thorough understanding of the physiology of vertebral subluxation and the vertebral adjustment. Through investigation of accepted scientific and physiological concepts, it has become increasingly evident that the interference in nerve impulse flow addressed by chiropractic can occur at locations other than the intervertebral foramen (IVF), although some of the ancillary effects of the adjustment may not be readily apparent.

Major points of this paper include the following:

- Chiropractic adjustments have been successful for almost a century.

- An objective of chiropractic is to achieve a purpose and to effect a change for the better.

- The majority of chiropractic patients experience symptomatic improvement from adjustments the majority of the time.

- Movement of vertebrae initiates far more extensive physiological responses than is generally recognized.

- Both the physiology of the adjustment and the physiology of subluxations have been explained in accepted scientific texts.

- A cause and effect relationship exists between structure and function.

- Chiropractic adjustments must be able to demonstrate structural changes for the better as well as symptomatic improvement.

- Any vertebral adjustment primarily affects the sensory nervous system. (Guyton p. 718)

- Approximately 99% of all incoming sensory information is discarded. (Guyton p. 609)

- Since 99% of sensory information is discarded, it follows that we are controlled 99% by memory engrams of past experiences, except in emergency, 1% becomes 100%.

- A subluxation may not be pathological since it represents a formerly appropriate vertebral position which is currently inappropriate for present need or intent.

- The position of vertebrae may be mandated by a memory engram that was imprinted when that particular vertebral position was necessary. (Guyton pp. 717)

- The Bio Energetic Synchronization Technique allows the subconscious to recognize that a malpositioned vertebra is no longer appropriate for present need.

- Subconscious areas of the central nervous system (principally in the thalamus-hypothalamus-cerebellum complex) are responsible for maintaining vertebral position.

- Bio Energetic Synchronization Technique allows the sensory system to update present physiology (vertebral position) to conform to present need or intent rather than to be influenced by compensated memory engrams.

- A vertebral adjustment may initiate a new engram which places the vertebra into a more normal position by way of indirect stimulation of the sensory system.

- Forceful adjustments signal the thalamus and lower areas of the brain indirectly by repositioning vertebrae.

- Vertebrae will sustain a new position when the new position is accepted as normal by the subconscious areas of the brain.

- Bio Energetic Synchronization Technique accomplishes vertebral repositioning by directly affecting the sensory system.

- Strong emotions can affect physiology. (Guyton p. 778)

- A memory engram pattern may dictate a response that is less than optimal due to a stress that was present when the engram was formed. (Guyton pp. 609, 610)

- Bio Energetic Synchronization Technique is a non-force procedure that will not precipitate a stress response.

- Vertebral adjustments may be diluted or compromised when adrenal stress response (fear, fight-flight) is initiated.

- Tactile stimulation or vertebral adjustment information will be stored if it is of sufficient intensity or duration to pose a threat to homeostasis.

- Afferent impulses from tactile stimulation or from vertebral adjustment pass to the subcortical areas of the brain — primarily the cerebellum — initiating efferent impulses that travel back to the muscles. (Guyton p. 660; Mountcastle pp. 1695, 1715)

- Bio Energetic Synchronization Technique utilizes light pressure on specific spinal, cephalic, and other body areas, which stimulates the initiation of a sensory response. (Mountcastle p. 1740)

- Five motor response body languages are employed in Bio Energetic Synchronization Technique analysis and therapy.

- Each of the five languages, vestibular, vision, respiration, kinesthetic, and somesthetic, communicates with a different level of the central nervous system. (Guyton pp. 696 ff., 755)

- Sensations as light as tactile pressure will elicit sensory signals both proximally and distally from the cerebellum. (Guyton p. 717; Mountcastle p. 1740)

- Muscle tension is responsible for bone position. (Guyton p. 685)

- Muscle receptors (muscle spindle and Golgi apparatus) apprise the sensorium of muscle length and tension and of joint position which, in turn, are stimulated by efferent impulses. (Guyton pp. 651, 660)

- Patient symptomatology is improved when the adjustment initiates sensory impulses that go to the brain and stimulate motor impulses that effect a change in muscle tone thereby allowing the new position to be sustained. (Guyton pp. 610, 685)

- The Bio Energetic Synchronization Technique accomplishes the chiropractic objective of vertebral repositioning.

- The Bio Energetic Synchronization Technique employs stress-free hands-only procedures to spinal areas that produce maximum benefit to the patient.

7

ADDENDUM

The Bio Energetic Synchronization Technique evolves continually. As additional information that has the potential to increase the power and comprehensive nature of the system becomes available, it is tested and either incorporated into the technique or, if it fails even once, it is discarded. The material that follows is just such information — information acquired and proved after the manuscript for this book went to the printer. I have found the concepts presented in this section to be of such significance that they now are an integral part of B.E.S.T. adjustments and included in my technique seminars.

An underlying theme of the B.E.S.T. system is that subluxations and disease are caused by present physiology that is the manifestation of responses to stimuli coming from memory. We have cited scientific literature indicating that 99% of the stimuli eliciting physiological responses come from memory.

On page 39, we discuss how the defense response can dilute the effectiveness of an adjustment and that the body attempts to preserve the vertebral position that existed before forceful repositioning. The patient's subconscious defense mechanism is so powerful that it can negate the physical force that was selected by the doctor's conscious mind. We have also seen throughout this study that conscious cortical activity is no match for subconscious responses. Unless the patient's memory patterns are updated to accept the new position, muscle spindle information along with the righting reflex can return the vertebra to its pre-adjustment position. It is important to understand that this defense mechanism exists and that the power it exerts on physical configuration can mean the difference between a successful and unsuccessful adjustment no matter what technique is used.

In this section, we will explain the concept of structural homeostasis and expand the concept of the defense response. We will also see how the adrenal response correlates with the musculoskeletal system and structural homeostasis.

DEFENSE REACTION

Chiropractic subscribes to the premise that the body is a self-healing, self-regulating entity, yet we know that even with the aid of adjustments, self-healing does not always take place. The subconscious that regulates both functional and structural homeostasis is non-judgmental — it makes repairs or corrections strictly on an on/off basis. The subconscious operates only in the here and now, neither planning for the future nor qualifying its responses. There is no "yes, but..." in subconscious reactions; mitigating circumstances are of no consequence to homeostasis.

Nowhere is this more obvious than in the defense response that alters the body's physiological functions, including muscle tone and posture, to gear the body for action. The defense response is either turned on or turned off. Both "on" and "off" are perfectly acceptable states for the body — they are both normal, appropriate conditions. Furthermore, the body does not differentiate between external stimuli and internal memory in activating the defense response. Defense physiology is always normal and appropriate to the stimulus, but the stimulus is not always appropriate to the current conditions or in the best interest of homeostasis. Stimuli from memory often bear little relationship to the needs of current conditions. For example, when a chance occurrence or remark triggers a memory of a similar past situation that was frightening or upsetting, the same anxiety that was elicited from the earlier experience will recur although no threat actually exists in the present scenario. Much of the 99% memory stimuli that influence physiology and dictate the defense response was created by anxiety. The conscious mind and subconscious mind of the patient have a profound effect on homeostasis in general and the recurring subluxation in particular — neither homeostatic changes nor health can be forced on anyone.

HOMEOSTASIS

To understand the impact of the defense response on health, we must recall that the human body constantly attempts to maintain optimum homeostasis. Depending upon the conditions imposed upon it, the state of equilibrium may or may not be ideal from the patient's physiological perspective. No matter how the body is functioning, it is moving toward equilibrium for the current situation.

Homeostasis is a vital, ongoing process that keeps the body in the best condition possible. It occurs without *thought*, governing the function of the many involuntary systems of the body, such as circulatory, respiratory, and organ function to name a few. It has become evident that homeostasis also monitors and controls structure. Structural homeostasis, or maintaining a steady-state equilibrium of structure, is just as vital to a patient's well-being as is functional homeostasis. Functional homeostasis and structural homeostasis occur without thought just as vertebral position is adopted without thought.

We have no muscles designed to pull bones out of position. Bones are positioned in accordance with homeostatic needs. Consequently, every position a vertebra can assume (with the exception of traumatically induced positions from accidents) is normal for that vertebra. Since it is a "normal" position, Innate

Intelligence does not recognize an apparent misalignment as abnormal, therefore will not correct it.

If vertebrae rotate and stay rotated, the individual has no conscious power over the muscles to pull the vertebrae back into proper position. Chiropractic has considered vertebral joints to be as freely moving as an elbow or knee joint. Joint receptors in communication with the cortex allow conscious control of elbow and knee joints. However, unlike elbows and knees, vertebrae cannot consciously be moved independently; we cannot decide to move our fifth dorsal independently of all other vertebrae.

The spine is an integrated, closed system. Force applied to any part of this closed system must be dissipated throughout the system. Cerebrospinal fluid is liquid in nature with minimal compression capabilities. Consequently, any external force applied to the vertebral column must be dispersed to other areas of the spine which may result in additional stress being inflicted at another location. In order to move one vertebra, adjoining vertebrae must also move, and this is accomplished most effectively by muscles. If stress is inflicted on one area of the spine, the defense response is activated and the stress will be absorbed and distributed equally throughout the unified spinal system.

CONSTITUENTS OF THE DEFENSE RESPONSE

Two components make up the physical aspects of the defense response: (1) the adrenal response, and (2) defense physiology, or skeletal muscle postural tone. Response patterns for both of these components are stored in the memory of each individual.

Adrenal Response

Guyton writes about the physical aspects of the adrenal response, or "Alarm" pattern, (7th edition, page 240, *Stimulation of the Hypothalamus — The 'Alarm' Pattern*) that includes increased blood supply to muscles and increased heart activity. "The arterial pressure rises, the cardiac output increases, the heart rate increases, and the circulation is ready to supply nutrients to the muscles if there be need. Also, impulses are transmitted simultaneously throughout the central nervous system to cause a state of generalized excitement and attentiveness, these often increasing to such a pitch that the overall pattern of the reaction is that of *alarm*, or sometimes also called the *defense pattern*."

Guyton also tell us (page 695, *'Alarm' or 'Stress' Response of the Sympathetic Nervous System*) that "The sympathetic system is also strongly activated in many emotional states. For instance, in the state of rage, which is elicited mainly by stimulating the hypothalamus...." In a previous section we saw how the pattern of this reaction can be stored in memory engrams and recalled as a response to a particular stimulus. A chiropractic adjustment that addresses a subluxation that is the effect of this memory pattern, without updating the memory, stands virtually no chance of holding after the patient sits up or stands. B.E.S.T. adjustments, on the other hand, focus on changing the stimulus that caused the subluxation to allow the muscles to respond and reposition vertebrae naturally.

Defense Physiology

Defense physiology incorporates functional, postural, and structural adaptations along with the adrenal response. In defense physiology — brought about by either an actual emergency or a perceived emergency such as anxiety — digestion is shut down, blood is directed to the skeletal muscles in anticipation of "battle," and muscles and skeletal position are primed for action. Most of the memory patterns that dictate a defense response were created by anxiety.

Defense physiology from memory affects:

(1) *function* that halts digestion and stimulates the adrenal response — the fight or flight reflex that, by our cultural standards, must be restrained or repressed,

(2) *posture* in a position adopted for defense — tight muscles that cannot be relaxed for an adjustment, and

(3) *structure* in positioning vertebrae — subluxations.

Defense physiology is normal. The manifestations of defense physiology are not subject to correction by Innate Intelligence. It is normal for the stomach to secrete acid, and it is also normal for the stomach not to secrete acid; it is normal for muscles to be tight, and it is also normal for muscles to be relaxed. None of these conditions, in and of themselves, needs to be "corrected" by Innate because none is an aberrant condition. However, Innate responds immediately, without conscious thought, to alter conditions when we touch a hot stove or step on a nail.

SKELETAL MUSCLES AND DEFENSE

There are three general types of muscles in the body:

- striated muscles = skeletal muscles

- cardiac muscles = heart muscles

- smooth muscles = visceral and multiunit smooth muscles

Skeletal muscles make up approximately 40% of the entire body while cardiac and smooth muscles make up approximately 10% (Guyton, page 120, *Contraction of Skeletal Muscle*). For the purpose of this study, our focus is on striated skeletal muscles.

Skeletal muscles attach to tendons that attach to bones; tendons create motion through muscle action. Even when healthy muscles are apparently relaxed, they are still slightly tense. Vertebrae are held in position by tone, or resting tension, of a striated muscle or group of muscles. Resting striated muscle tone is controlled subconsciously by:

(1) the muscle spindle in the belly of the striated muscle that determines muscle length, and

(2) the Golgi tendon organ that determines muscle tension.

Muscle spindles and Golgi organs transmit signals pertaining to muscle length and tension to the cerebellum — a part of the subconscious nervous system — and we are aware of vertebral muscle tension only at the subconscious level which explains why we can consciously relax back muscles only to a limited degree. Since 99% of physiology is governed subconsciously by stimuli coming from memory, muscular tenseness can be precipitated and maintained by this defensive stored memory. The subconscious nature of muscle tenseness is apparent to chiropractors when patients claim to be completely relaxed on the adjusting table yet palpation shows specific muscle groups to be tightly contracted. It is this subconscious tension that sets the stage for inappropriate homeostatic structure that is called a subluxation.

Structural homeostasis occurs without thought, consequently, vertebral position occurs without thought. All of the body, including structure, responds only on a stimulus-response level. When the adrenal response is elicited by either an external or internal stimulus, including a chiropractic adjustment, muscle tension along with other subconscious reactions respond.

All chiropractic adjustments can update engrams of past experience and replace the defense response stored in memory with patterns consistent with current need. The defense posture for fight or flight is sometimes appropriate, but only as a short-term condition. When this response is retained over long periods, both functional homeostasis and structural homeostasis become physiologically destructive as exhaustion occurs. The physiological processes necessary to protect the body when it is threatened are emergency measures. When survival is the priority of the body, growth and replenishment become secondary. Hard, forceful chiropractic adjustments under these conditions may not be sustained and may cause additional stress to the body thus exacerbating the defense reaction.

The ideal adjustment does not elicit a defense response, however three primary factors can influence the effectiveness of any chiropractic adjustment:

(1) the function of all living systems is directed toward normalcy;

(2) muscle spindles and Golgi organs relay information to the cerebellum (subcortical) which controls all musculoskeletal coordination; and

(3) the defense response can be elicited.

If an attempt is made to move vertebrae while a patient is responding to a memory-generated stimulus that has prompted defensive physiology, the subconscious of that patient will respond to the need for additional defense and maintain the muscle tenseness despite the patient's conscious attempt to relax the muscles.

Although misaligned vertebrae and tense muscles may exist at an inappropriate time, the body will not attempt to correct that which is normal for some experience. Recall that bone cannot move into a position that is not normal, except through trauma. A vertebra that appears on an x-ray to be subluxated is in reality maintaining a quite proper position for a different posture. The position is not wrong, but it is no longer appropriate for the prevailing circumstances.

The only way to alleviate the results of a response precipitated by a memory stimulus is to update the stimulus to conform to non-emergency conditions that currently exist. This is done by helping the subconscious to become aware of the current situation. Passive manipulation of the muscles through a range of motion allows the muscle spindles to associate the position with non-stressful, pleasant mental images and appropriate patterns to be stored in memory. When the pleasant experience is recalled, the defense posture can be nullified since defense physiology is not appropriate for pleasant experiences.

We communicate with the subconscious primarily through sight, hearing, and touch. Most of our pleasant experiences provide sensations associated with one of these; however, experiences that arouse a pleasurable response in one person will not necessarily have the same effect on everyone. A patient who was having trouble relaxing was asked if he had ever been to the ocean. He replied that he had, but when he was asked if that experience was pleasant and relaxing, he responded that he found the ocean terrifying. Certainly, encouraging this patient to visualize his experience will not move him out of his defensive posture. However, an experience that he finds pleasing will allow his muscles to relax.

Treatment with non-threatening, non-traumatic therapeutic adjustments of B.E.S.T. can allow more appropriate information to be stored in memory. With this revised information, the health-restoring internal environment will allow the body to repair itself in the way nature intended.

APPENDIX A

REPRODUCTIONS OF PRE-TREATMENT AND POST-TREATMENT X-RAYS AND CAT SCAN REPORT ILLUSTRATING STRUCTURAL IMPROVEMENT OF PATIENTS THROUGH ADJUSTMENTS USING THE BIO ENERGETIC SYNCHRONIZATION TECHNIQUE

The following photographs showing "Before" and "After" x-rays and CAT Scan report demonstrate that the Bio Energetic Synchronization Technique has a beneficial effect on the structure-function relationship that is achieved by the body's own inner laws acting to regulate structure and function.

Notice that in some pictures the body may appear to have over-corrected in one area of the spine as a correction is occurring in the other end of the spine.

The only chiropractic technique used on these patients was the Bio Energetic Synchronization Technique. No lifts were used.

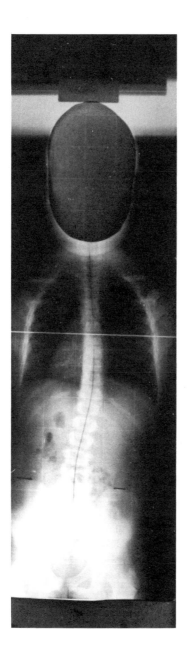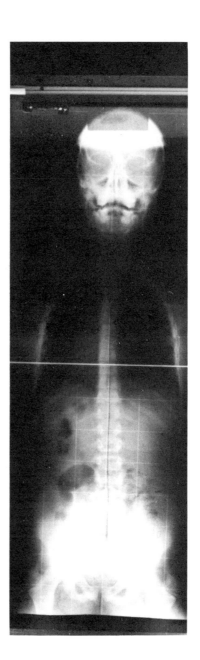

Ten year old male. Major complaints: right foot pain, leg pain, neck pain, shoulder pain as result of boating accident. Duration of symptoms prior to treatment, "few weeks." Had consulted several M.D.'s. Course of care 6 months. Patient comment upon dismissal: "Feeling great."

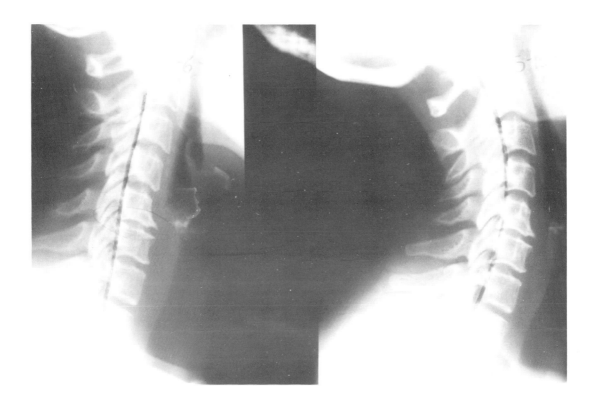

Forty year old female; registered nurse. Major complaints: neck pain, upper back
pain, hip pain, knee pain. Cause of symptoms, insidious; duration of symptoms
"years." Patient had consulted other D.C.'s. Course of care: 5 weeks. Patient comment: "Much better."

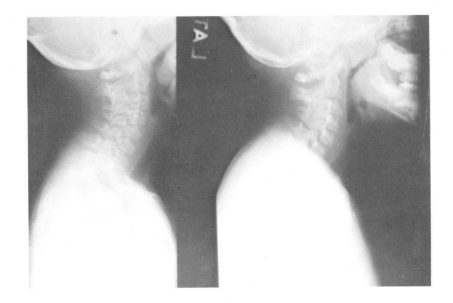

Neutral

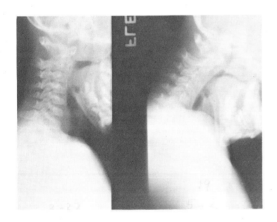

Flexion

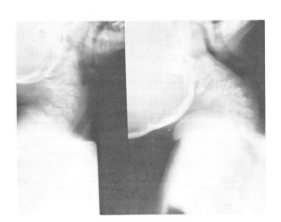

Extension

Five year old female complaining of neck pain and mid-back pain following automobile accident. Duration of symptoms prior to treatment, 2 days. Patient had not consulted other doctors. Course of care, 5 weeks. Patient comment: "Feeling great."

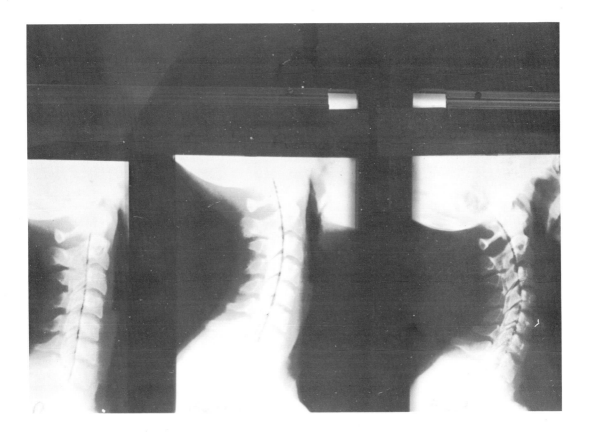

Twenty-two year old female. Occupation: secretary. Major complaints low-back, mid-back, neck pain, headaches. Cause unknown. Duration of symptoms had been 2 weeks; course of care 3 months. Patient had not been treated by other doctors. Patient comment , "Much better."

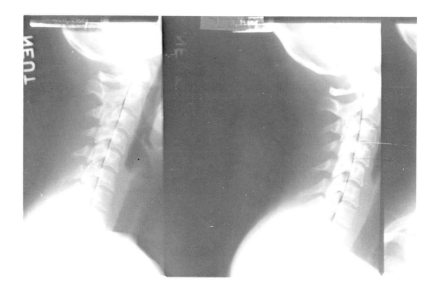

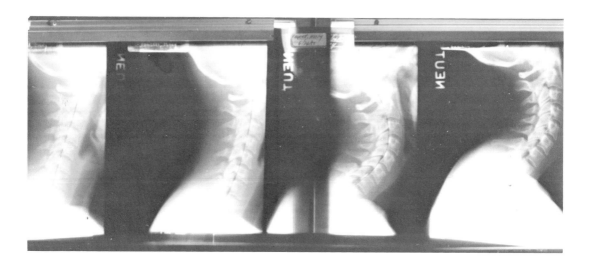

Twenty-four year old female. Occupation: secretary. Complained of neck, back pain, right hip pain, left calf pain, cause unknown. Duration of symptoms before treatment 2 weeks. Course of care 6 months. This patient had not consulted other doctors. Patient comment, "Much better."

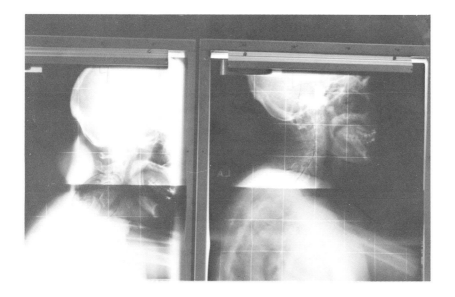

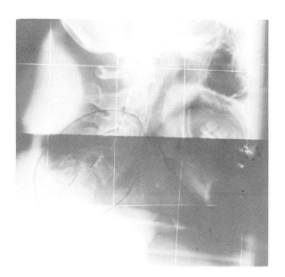
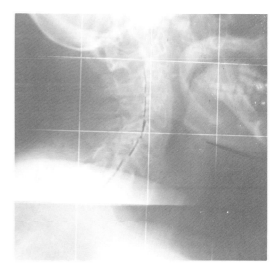

Seventy-nine year old retired female complained of mid-back pain, side pain, occasional low-back pain resulting from a fall. Pain had persisted for 4 months during which time she had been treated by other D.C.'s. Course of care was 5 weeks. Patient comment upon dismissal — "Feeling great."

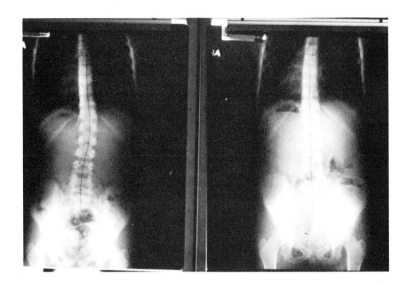

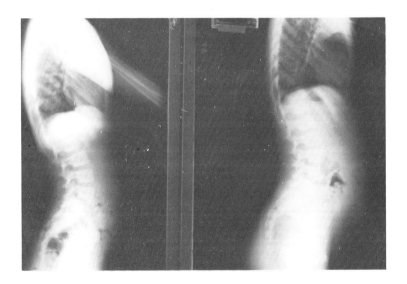

Seven year old female complained of neck pain and low-back pain as the result of an automobile accident. Symptoms had persisted for two weeks prior to initial treatment. Duration of chiropractic care was 3 months. This patient had not been treated by other doctors. Patient comment upon dismissal — "Feeling great."

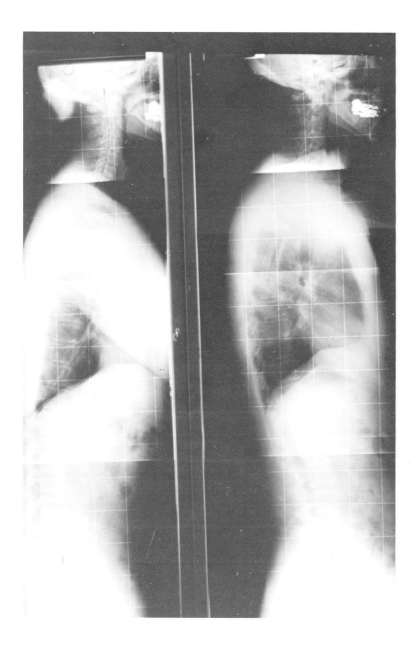

Fifty year old male; occupation: sales. Major complaints: low-back pain, hip pain after lifting lawn mower out of trunk of car. Duration of symptoms: "a few days." Patient had consulted several other D.C.'s. Course of care, 5 weeks. Patient comment upon dismissal, "Feeling great."

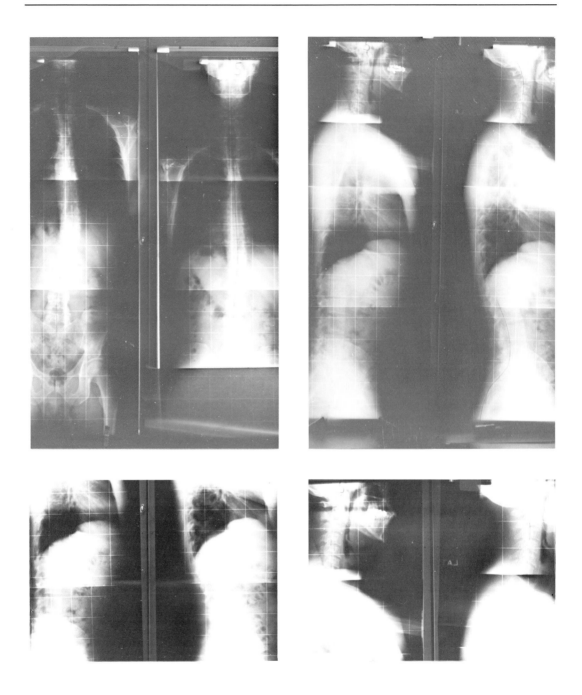

Thirty-nine year old male; occupation: coal handler. Complaints included low-back pain, leg pain, hip pain, and headaches attributed to unloading wood. Duration of symptoms before treatment, 2 days. Course of care: 1 month. Patient comment upon dismissal, "Feeling great."

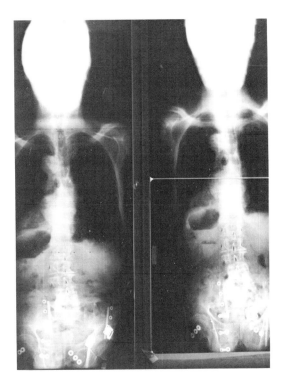

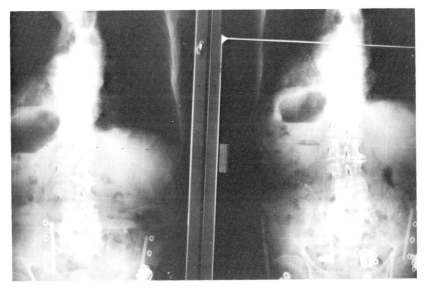

Eighty-nine year old male, retired. Major complaints: low-back pain, leg pain, foot pain, neck pain following fall. Duration of symptoms had been 1 month. Course of care 7 weeks. Patient had not been treated by other doctors. Patient comment: "Better."

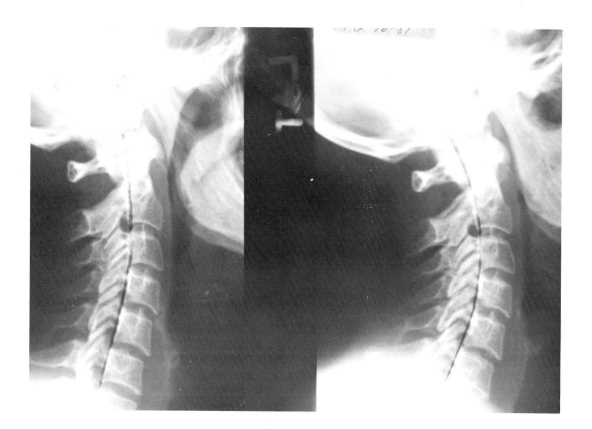

Thirty-nine year old female; housewife. Major complaints: headaches, neck pain, mid-back pain, nausea. Duration of symptoms, several (10) years. Cause: insidious. Patient had consulted M.D., Neurologist, had 2 CAT scans, 2 EEG's, and Venous Arteriogram. Course of care 3 weeks. Patient comment: "Much better."

CAT SCAN REPORT

Herniated Disc

History: 30-year old female nursing home employee, weight 215 lbs., height 5' 7", presented complaining of low back pain from a traumatically induced injury. The patient further explained that she twisted and felt her back pop while lifting a patient from a bed to a chair, and experienced instant pain. CAT scan revealed "lateral herniated disc that is present and entrapping nerve root in the L 4–5 foramen on the left side." This report was written by a local orthopedic surgeon, M.D., who reviewed the CAT scans performed at a local hospital.

The patient was treated with Bio Energetic Synchronization Technique for approximately 12 weeks. Pre- and post-treatment thermographic evaluations indicate a marked reduction in symptom complex. Patient has shown complete recovery without surgery and is presently asymptomatic.

APPENDIX B

LABORATORY ANALYSIS COMPARISONS

REPRODUCTIONS OF PATIENT BLOOD PROFILES

The following blood profile data from laboratory reports demonstrate the positive effect the Bio Energetic Synchronization system has on toxicity and homeostasis of the patient.

BLOOD PROFILE

Patient: "A"

Patient Age and Sex: 30 year old Female

Date of: Test 1: 1-13-86   Test 2: 2-14-86

	Test 1: 1-13-86	Test 2: 2-14-86
HDL Cholesterol	38 mg/dl	26 mg/dl
Osmolality, Calculated	300 mosm/kg	286 mosm/kg
BUN/Creatinine Ratio	10	17
LDL Cholesterol, Calculated	121 mg/dl	142 mg/dl
CHD Risk	1.29 times average (Normal=1.0)	1.20 times average
VLDL Cholesterol (Calculated)	30 mg/dl	16 mg/dl

	Test 1	Test 2
BONE		
Calcium mg/dl (8.5-10.6)	9.6	9.4
Phosphorus mg/dl (2.5-4.5)	3.9	2.6
ELECTROLYTES		
Sodium mEq/L (135-148)	147	139
Potassium mEq/L (3.5-5.5)	4.2	4.0
Chloride mEq/L (94-109)	103	101
HEART		
LDH IU/L (100-250)	276 High	228
SGOT IU/L (0-50)	132 High	83 High
LIVER		
T.Bili mg/dl (0.1-1.2)	0.3	0.4
GGT (IU/L) (M 0-65) (F 0-45)	29	30
SGPT IU/L (0-50)	73 High	106 High
Alk. Phos. IU/L (20-125)	106	103
LIPIDS		
Cholesterol mg/dl (115-295)	189	185
Triglycerides mg/dl (10-190)	150	83
PROTEIN		
T. Protein g/dl (6.0-8.5)	7.7	7.6
Globulin g/dl (1.5-4.5)	3.2	3.0
Albumin g/dl (3.5-5.5)	4.5	4.6
A/G Ratio g/dl (1.1-2.5)	1.4	1.5
KIDNEY		
BUN mg/dl (7-26)	9	12
Creatinine mg/dl (0.5-1.5)	0.9	0.7
THYROID		
T_4 μg/dl (4.5-12.5)	7.2	9.3
T_3 Uptake % (35-45)	32 Low	32 Low
Free T_4 Index (1.6-5.6)	2.3	2.9
TSH μIU/ml (<5.0)	—	—

	Test 1	Test 2
MISCELLANEOUS		
Uric Acid mg/dl (M 3.9-9.0) (F 2.2-7.7)	6.9	8.1 High
Glucose mg/dl <50 yrs (60-115)	64	83
Iron μg/dl (40-180)	—	—
HEMATOLOGY		
RBC x 10⁶/mm³ (M 4.3-5.9) (F 3.5-5.5)	4.65	4.45
HGB g/dl (M 13.9-18.0) (F 12.0-16.0)	15.0	14.5
HCT % (M 39-55) (F 36-48)	44.7	42.9
MCV μ³ (80-100)	96	96
MCH μμg (26-34)	32.2	32.5
MCHC % (31-37)	33.5	33.7
Platelets x 10³/mm³ (150-500)	ADQ	ADQ
WBC x 10³/mm³ (4.0-10.5)	11.8 High	8.3
Polys (45-75%) (1.5-8.0)	66	62
Absolute Value:	7.4	4.9
Bands (0-5%)	—	—
Absolute Value: Metas (0%)	—	—
Absolute Value: Lymphs (20-45%) (0.8-3.2)	28	32
Absolute Value:	3.4H	2.6
Mono (0-10%) (0-0.5)	4	2
Absolute Value:	0.5	0.2
EOS (0-6%) (0-0.5)	2	4
Absolute Value:	0.2	0.3
BASO (0-2%) (0-0.1)	0	0
Absolute Value	0.0	0.0

BLOOD PROFILE

Patient: "B"
Patient Age and Sex: 31 year old Female

Date of:	Test 1: 8-1-86	Test 2: 6-29-87
HDL Cholesterol	37 mg/dl	32 mg/dl
Osmolality, Calculated	290 mosm/kg	292 mosm/kg
BUN/Creatinine Ratio	12	8
LDL Cholesterol, Calculated	135 mg/dl	119 mg/dl
CHD Risk	1.50 times average	1.20 times average
VLDL Cholesterol (Calculated)	29 mg/dl	30 mg/dl

	Test 1	Test 2
BONE		
Calcium mg/dl (8.5-10.6)	9.6	9.8
Phosphorus mg/dl (2.5-4.5)	2.8	4.1
ELECTROLYTES		
Sodium mEq/L (135-148)	141	143
Potassium mEq/L (3.5-5.5)	4.2	4.4
Chloride mEq/L (94-109)	103	104
HEART		
LDH IU/L (100-250)	195	156
SGOT IU/L (0-50)	74 High	36
LIVER		
T.Bili mg/dl (0.1-1.2)	0.3	0.2
GGT (IU/L) (M 0-65) (F 0-45)	29	19
SGPT IU/L (0-50)	76 High	43
Alk. Phos. IU/L (20-125)	110	105
LIPIDS		
Cholesterol mg/dl (115-295)	202	182
Triglycerides mg/dl (10-190)	149	151
PROTEIN		
T. Protein g/dl (6.0-8.5)	7.5	7.5
Globulin g/dl (1.5-4.5)	3.1	2.8
Albumin g/dl (3.5-5.5)	4.4	4.7
A/G Ratio g/dl (1.1-2.5)	1.4	1.6
KIDNEY		
BUN mg/dl (7-26)	9	6 Low
Creatinine mg/dl (0.5-1.5)	0.7	0.7
THYROID		
T_4 μg/dl (4.5-12.5)	7.6	8.6
T_3 Uptake % (35-45)	34 Low	30 Low
Free T_4 Index (1.6-5.6)	2.5	2.5
TSH μIU/ml (<5.0)	—	—

	Test 1	Test 2
MISCELLANEOUS		
Uric Acid mg/dl		
(M 3.9-9.0) (F 2.2-7.7)	7.2	6.6
Glucose mg/dl <50 yrs		
(60-115)	100	91
Iron μg/dl (40-180)	—	—
HEMATOLOGY		
RBC x 10^6/mm^3		
(M 4.3-5.9) (F 3.5-5.5)	4.81	4.46
HGB g/dl		
(M 13.9-18.0) (F 12.0-16.0)	15.6	14.5
HCT % (M 39-55) (F 36-48)	46.6	42.5
MCV μ^3 (80-100)	96	95
MCH μμg (26-34)	32.4	32.6
MCHC % (31-37)	33.5	34.2
Platelets x 10^3/mm^3		
(150-500)	ADQ	250
WBC x 10^3/mm^3 (4.0-10.5)	9.0	10.3
Polys (45-75%) (1.5-8.0)	63	60
Absolute Value:	5.4	6.0
Bands (0-5%)	—	—
Absolute Value:		
Metas (0%)	—	—
Absolute Value:		
Lymphs (20-45%) (0.8-3.2)	28	36
Absolute Value:	2.5	3.7 H
Mono (0-10%) (0-0.5)	5	2
Absolute Value:	0.4	0.3
EOS (0-6%) (0-0.5)	4	2
Absolute Value:	0.3	0.2
BASO (0-2%) (0-0.1)	0	0
Absolute Value	0.0	0.0

BLOOD PROFILE

Patient: "C"

Patient Age and Sex: 56 year old Male

Date of: Test 1: 4-6-87   Test 2: 5-20-87

	Test 1	Test 2
HDL Cholesterol	30 mg/dl	29 mg/dl
Osmolality, Calculated	286 mosm/kg	294 mosm/kg
BUN/Creatinine Ratio	15	12
LDL Cholesterol, Calculated	Triglyceride result too high for accurate Beta cholesterol estimation	111 mg/dl
CHD Risk	1.40 times average (Normal=1.0)	1.16 times average
VLDL Cholesterol (Calculated)	Calculation not valid when triglyceride level is greater than 400 mg/dl	48 H mg/dl

	Test 1	Test 2
BONE		
Calcium mg/dl (8.5-10.6)	9.4	9.3
Phosphorus mg/dl (2.5-4.5)	3.2	2.7
ELECTROLYTES		
Sodium mEq/L (135-148)	139	143
Potassium mEq/L (3.5-5.5)	4.2	4.6
Chloride mEq/L (94-109)	102	106
HEART		
LDH IU/L (100-250)	137	129
SGOT IU/L (0-50)	55 High	69 High
LIVER		
T.Bili mg/dl (0.1-1.2)	0.4	0.4
GGT (IU/L) (M 0-65) (F 0-45)	31	35
SGPT IU/L (0-50)	54 High	62 High
Alk. Phos. IU/L (20-125)	49	62
LIPIDS		
Cholesterol mg/dl (115-295)	213	189
Triglycerides mg/dl (10-190)	528 High	241 High
PROTEIN		
T. Protein g/dl (6.0-8.5)	7.6	7.5
Globulin g/dl (1.5-4.5)	3.5	3.0
Albumin g/dl (3.5-5.5)	4.1	4.5
A/G Ratio g/dl (1.1-2.5)	1.1	1.5
KIDNEY		
BUN mg/dl (7-26)	14	12
Creatinine mg/dl (0.5-1.5)	0.9	1.0
THYROID		
T_4 μg/dl (4.5-12.5)	5.2	7.1
T_3 Uptake % (35-45)	32 Low	31 Low
Free T_4 Index (1.6-5.6)	1.6	2.2
TSH μIU/ml (<5.0)	—	—

	Test 1	Test 2
MISCELLANEOUS		
Uric Acid mg/dl (M 3.9-9.0) (F 2.2-7.7)	6.1	6.6
Glucose mg/dl <50 yrs (60-115)	85	92
Iron μg/dl (40-180)	—	—
HEMATOLOGY		
RBC x 10⁶/mm³ (M 4.3-5.9) (F 3.5-5.5)	5.16	5.26
HGB g/dl (M 13.9-18.0) (F 12.0-16.0)	16.5	16.4
HCT % (M 39-55) (F 36-48)	48.2	47.9
MCV μ³ (80-100)	93	91
MCH μμg (26-34)	32.0	31.2
MCHC % (31-37)	34.3	34.3
Platelets x 10³/mm³ (150-500)	232	238
WBC x 10³/mm³ (4.0-10.5)	9.2	6.5
Polys (45-75%) (1.5-8.0)	52	51
Absolute Value:	4.6	3.1
Bands (0-5%)	—	—
Absolute Value:		
Metas (0%)	—	—
Absolute Value:		
Lymphs (20-45%) (0.8-3.2)	39	41
Absolute Value:	3.5 H	2.7
Mono (0-10%) (0-0.5)	—	—
Absolute Value:		
EOS (0-6%) (0-0.5)	2	2
Absolute Value:	0.2	0.1
BASO (0-2%) (0-0.1)	2	2
Absolute Value:	0.2	0.1

Calcium

$RBC \times 10^6/mm^3$

BLOOD PROFILE

Patient: "D"
Patient Age and Sex: 16 year old Male

Date of:	Test 1: 8-19-86	Test 2: 8-26-86
HDL Cholesterol	45 mg/dl	71 mg/dl
Osmolality, Calculated	287 mosm/kg	282 mosm/kg
BUN/Creatinine Ratio	13	10
LDL Cholesterol, Calculated	94 mg/dl	77 mg/dl
CHD Risk	0.60 times average (Normal=1.0)	0.24 times average
VLDL Cholesterol (Calculated)	22 mg/dl	34 mg/dl

	Test 1	Test 2
BONE		
Calcium mg/dl (8.5-10.6)	9.6	9.9
Phosphorus mg/dl (2.5-4.5)	3.3	3.3
ELECTROLYTES		
Sodium mEq/L (135-148)	139	138
Potassium mEq/L (3.5-5.5)	4.8	4.6
Chloride mEq/L (94-109)	101	99
HEART		
LDH IU/L (100-250)	292 High	155
SGOT IU/L (0-50)	152 High	33
LIVER		
T.Bili mg/dl (0.1-1.2)	0.5	0.3
GGT (IU/L) (M 0-65) (F 0-45)	15	12
SGPT IU/L (0-50)	70 High	26
Alk. Phos. IU/L (20-125)	195	151
LIPIDS		
Cholesterol mg/dl (115-295)	161	182
Triglycerides mg/dl (10-190)	110	170
PROTEIN		
T. Protein g/dl (6.0-8.5)	7.4	6.6
Globulin g/dl (1.5-4.5)	3.0	2.4
Albumin g/dl (3.5-5.5)	4.4	4.2
A/G Ratio g/dl (1.1-2.5)	1.4	1.7
KIDNEY		
BUN mg/dl (7-26)	13	8
Creatinine mg/dl (0.5-1.5)	1.0	0.8
THYROID		
T_4 µg/dl (4.5-12.5)	7.6	6.6
T_3 Uptake % (35-45)	37	35
Free T_4 Index (1.6-5.6)	2.8	2.3
TSH µIU/ml (<5.0)	—	—

	Test 1	Test 2
MISCELLANEOUS		
Uric Acid mg/dl (M 3.9-9.0) (F 2.2-7.7)	6.6	6.0
Glucose mg/dl <50 yrs (60-115)	95	85
Iron µg/dl (40-180)	—	—
HEMATOLOGY		
RBC x 10^6/mm³ (M 4.3-5.9) (F 3.5-5.5)	5.22	5.56
HGB g/dl (M 13.9-18.0) (F 12.0-16.0)	15.5	16.3
HCT % (M 39-55) (F 36-48)	46.8	50.5
MCV µ³ (80-100)	89	90
MCH µµg (26-34)	29.7	29.4
MCHC % (31-37)	33.1	32.4
Platelets x 10³/mm³ (150-500)	248	218
WBC x 10³/mm³ (4.0-10.5)	10.0	6.3
Polys (45-75%) (1.5-8.0)	77 H	67
Absolute Value:	7.5	4.1
Bands (0-5%)	—	—
Absolute Value:		
Metas (0%)	—	—
Absolute Value:		
Lymphs (20-45%) (0.8-3.2)	14 L	27
Absolute Value:	1.4	1.7
Mono (0-10%) (0-0.5)	7	4
Absolute Value:	0.7	0.2
EOS (0-6%) (0-0.5)	2	2
Absolute Value:	0.2	0.1
BASO (0-2%) (0-0.1)	0	0
Absolute Value:	0.0	0.0

BIOGRAPHY

M.T. MORTER, JR., B.S., M.A., D.C.

M.T. Morter, Jr., earned his Bachelor of Science degree from Kent State University, Kent, Ohio. He was awarded a Master of Arts in Science Education from Ohio State University, and a Doctor of Chiropractic from Logan College of Chiropractic in St. Louis. He holds professional licenses in the states of Arkansas, Missouri, Colorado, Texas and Indiana.

Prior to entering the profession of chiropractic, Dr. Morter was in the field of education teaching science and mathematics at the secondary level.

Dr. Morter has been in private practice since 1965, during which time he established Morter Chiropractic Clinic in Rogers, Arkansas. The clinic staff has grown to keep pace with the increasing patient volume and now includes nine D.C.'s in addition to Dr. Morter.

Dr. Morter continues to be heavily involved in education along with maintaining his patient commitments and clinic responsibilities. He has served as president of both Logan College of Chiropractic in St. Louis and Parker College of Chiropractic in Dallas, and, as a member of the associate faculties of both Logan College and Texas College, he has taught Chiropractic Philosophy, Technique, and Nutrition at both the undergraduate and graduate levels. In addition, he has been actively involved in professional organizations at the state and national levels, including:

Arkansas Chiropractic Association

- Board of Directors
- Second Vice-President
- Student Recruitment
- Legal Affairs and Legislative Committee
- Peer Review Guidelines Committee
- Grievance Committee
- Scientific and Educational Research
- Inter-Professional Committee
- Membership Committee

Council of Chiropractic Education

- Research Committee
- Specialty Councils Committee
- Auxiliary Sponsorship Committee
- Post Graduate and Related Professional Education Committee

Council of College Presidents

Secretary of Council

Dr. Morter has spoken before many institutions and organizations.

Convention Speaking Engagements

- Logan College
- Wisconsin State Convention
- Southeast Missouri Chiropractic Association
- New York State Association Convention
- Northwest Ohio Chiropractic Association
- Ohio State Convention
- Parker Seminar
- Illinois State Convention
- North Carolina State Convention

- *Texas State Convention
- *Missouri State Convention
- *Kansas State Convention
- *Texas Chiropractic College Convention
- Academy for Research in Chiropractic Sciences International
- National Academy of Research Biochemists
- *Arkansas State Convention
- *Georgia State Convention

Guest Speaking Engagements

- Hypoglycemia Society, Bettendorf, Iowa
- Cancer Prevention, Rogers, Arkansas
- Nutrition, St. Louis, Missouri
- Your Mind Matters, Kansas City, Missouri
- Your Split Second of Perfection, Dallas, Texas
- Improve Your Life, St. Louis, Missouri
- Innate - Friend or Foe?, Palmer Chiropractic College
- Innate and the Gall Bladder, Palmer Chiropractic College

He conducts continuing education seminars on Bio Energetic Synchronization Technique and nutrition throughout the United States and abroad and acts as consultant to other members of the profession. Seminar locations have included:

Joplin, Missouri
Dallas, Texas
Lowellsville, Ohio
Little Rock, Arkansas
Montreal, Quebec
Phoenix, Arizona
St. Louis, Missouri
Columbus, Ohio
Maui, Hawaii
Clearwater, Florida
Kansas City, Missouri
Baton Rouge, Louisiana
Eu Claire, Wisconsin
Toronto, Ontario
Daytona Beach, Florida
Los Angeles, California
Davenport, Iowa

Melbourne, Australia
Atlanta, Georgia
Chicago, Illinois
Perth, Australia
Capetown, South Africa
Rogers, Arkansas
New York, New York
San Francisco, California
Fayetteville, Arkansas
Toledo, Ohio
Charlotte, North Carolina
Orlando, Florida
* Eureka Springs, Arkansas

* License Renewal

Since 1975, Dr. Morter's articles have frequently been published in professional publications, and he and his work have been featured in the *St. Louis Magazine*, *American Chiropractor*, *Today's Chirporactic*, and *WorldWide Report*. His publications have appeared in:

> *Chiropractic Economics*
>
> *Today's Chiropractic*
>
> *The American Chiropractor*
>
> *The Chiropractic Professional*

Prior to the incidents that led to the development of the Bio Energetic Synchronization Technique, Dr. Morter practiced Basic, Gonstead, and Applied Kinesiology techniques. The Bio Energetic Synchronization Technique syllabus has been approved through Logan College of Chiropractic, Texas Chiropractic College, Life College of Chiropractic — West and Parker College of Chiropractic. Dr. Morter currently holds Adjunct Professor status through Texas Chiropractic College.

Dr. Morter lives in Rogers, Arkansas, with his wife, Marjorie Kibler Morter. Their three children, M.T. Morter, III, M. Thomas Morter, and Patricia Sue Morter are all Doctors of Chiropractic.

The order form below is provided for your convenience in obtaining additional copies of Chiropractic Physiology for yourself, your friends, or associates.

BEST RESEARCH, INC.
1000 W. Poplar
Rogers, AR 72756

Please send _____ copies of Chiropractic Physiology to me at the

address below. Enclosed is $_____

Name _____
Print or Type

Mailing Address _____

_____

_____

Cost per copy: $32.00 plus $3 postage and handling